Bristol
Medico-Historical
Society

PROCEEDINGS

Volume Seven

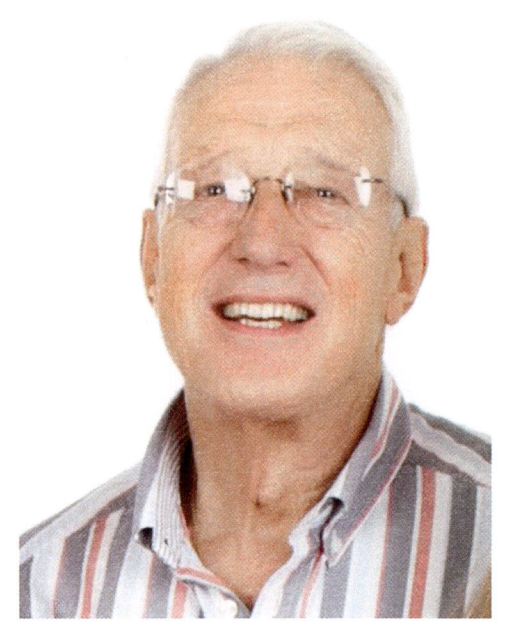

Bruno Bubna-Kastelitz
SEVENTH PRESIDENT OF THE SOCIETY

Bristol
Medico-Historical
Society

PROCEEDINGS

Volume Seven

Edited by

Paul R Goddard

MMXVI

Published by the **Bristol Medico-Historical Society**
Redland Green Farm
Redland
Bristol
BS6 7HF
© **Bristol Medico-Historical Society** 2016

First published in the UK 2016

ISBN 978-1-85457-090-1

Published by: Clinical Press Ltd for **Bristol Medico-Historical Society**

Redland Green Farm, Redland, Bristol, BS6 7HF, UK.

Contents

Frontispiece, Bruno Bubna-Kasteliz...seventh president of the society

Obituary: Beryl Corner	Peter M. Dunn	1
Nutrition and the Death Camps	Stella Dilke	10
Medical Aspects of the Younghusband Mission to Tibet	Vincent Marmion	36
Medical Fraud- Causes and Consequences	Gordon M. Stirrat	41
The Junior Doctors' Dispute 1975	Paul R. Goddard	51
Francis Galton- A passion for measurement	Martin Crosfill	62
The first Medical Missionary to India	Mike Whitfield	76
A History of ECT	Peter Carpenter	84
Fin-de-siècle: male hysteria	Tom Nutting	89
Edith and Florence Stoney, X-ray pioneers	Francis Duck	90
Fetal Compression and Congenital Deformation	Peter M. Dunn	99
Lessons from Royal Operations:	Walford Gillison	113
A Short history of Old Age Pensions	Bruno Bubna-Kasteliz	129
A history of Inebriacy in Bristol	Peter Carpenter	142
The Rise and Fall of Childbed Fever	Peter M. Dunn	151
The Pill and the Pope	Thomas F. Baskett	165
The Public Health of Victorian Bristol: Unhealthy Bristol	Peter Malpass	179
The Bristol Medico-Historical Society Programme	2012-2016	191

OBITUARY:

Beryl Corner
OBE, JP, MD, FRCP (Lond),FRCPCh (Hon),
MD Hon (Bristol), DSc Hon (UWE)
(1910 – 2007)

PETER M. DUNN, MA, MD, FRCP, FRCOG, FRCPCH
Professor Emeritus of Perinatal Medicine & Child Health
University of Bristol, Southmead Hospital
e-mail: P.M.Dunn@bristol.ac.uk

Beryl Corner was a founder member of the Bristol Medico-Historical Society in 1985 and its third President, 1995-1999. Many of you will remember her contributions to our Proceedings which included papers on *'The Care of the Newborn in Antiquity'* and *'The Beginning of Neonatology in Bristol'*. She also spoke to us about Dr. Elizabeth Blackwell and Clemens Von Pirquet. In her last talk at the age of 94 in 2004, she gave us a memorable account of the bombing of the Bristol Children's Hospital in 1942: *'Phoenix arises from the Ashes'*. Beryl died following a stroke in March 2007 at the age of 96. I had the privilege of giving an address at her thanksgiving service in Christchurch, Clifton. In the very short time available today, I think it best if I repeat what I said on that occasion:

'As a paediatrician, I was a colleague of Dr. Beryl Corner at Southmead Hospital from 1963 onwards. Beryl's nieces from America, Jane and Sally, have asked me to say a few words about Dr. Corner's professional career. This is some task! How does one compress into a few minutes Beryl's achievements during 42 years of active medical practice, followed by another 30 years of almost equally active retirement? Many, including myself, have always regarded Beryl as being indestructible. Maybe we were not wrong, for she has left us with memories that will remain fresh for many, many years to come.'

Beryl was born in Henleaze, Bristol, on December 9th, 1910, and received her education at Redland High School for Girls where she was regularly placed top of the form. She began her medical training at the Royal Free Hospital in London with the aid of a scholarship at the age of 17 (Fig 1).

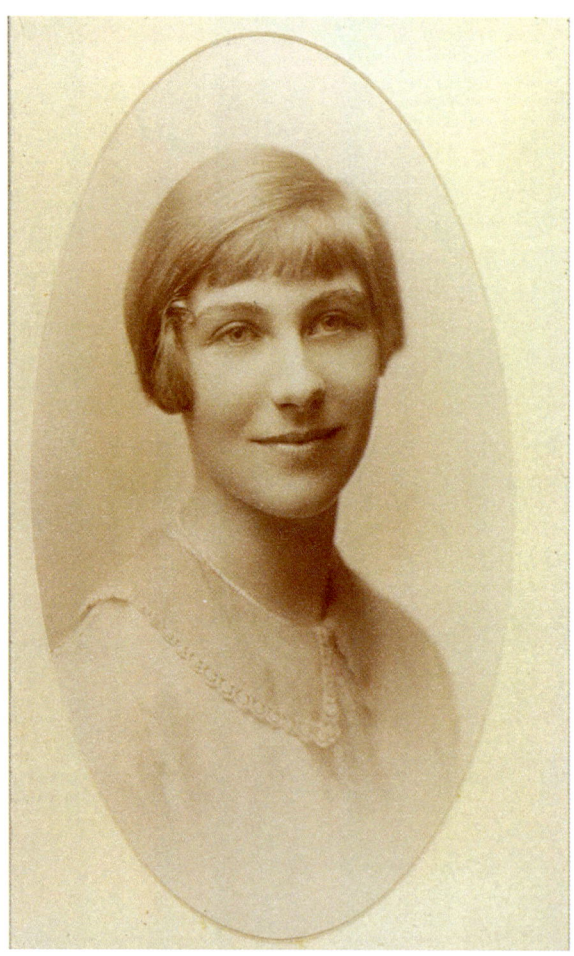

Fig 1 Beryl Corner, aged 17

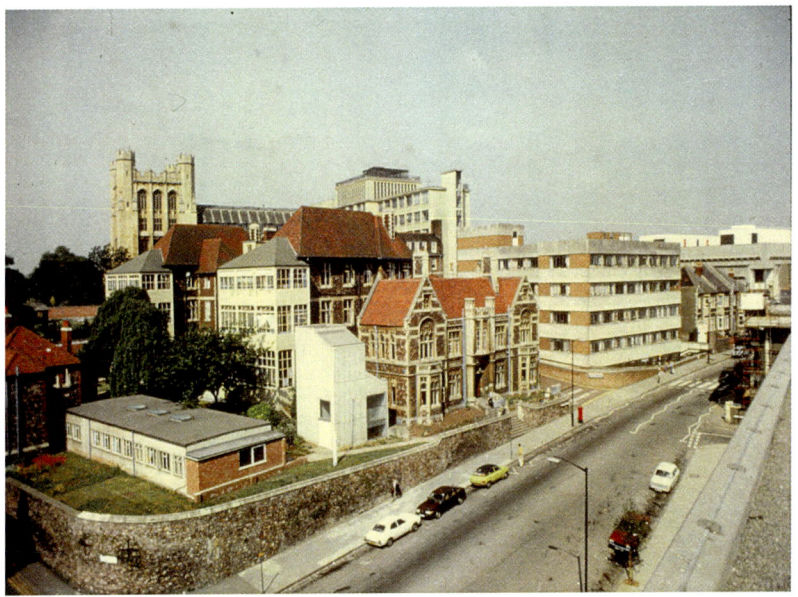

Fig 2 Royal Hospital for Sick Children, Bristol, 1990

She was a brilliant student, winning prizes in no less than five clinical subjects. Qualifying as a doctor in 1934, she then acquired both an MD and an MRCP within the next two years, and at the age of twenty-six was appointed Honorary Physician to the Out-Patients at the Royal Hospital for Sick Children, here in Bristol, thus becoming the first paediatrician to be appointed in the South West of England (Fig 2).

During the years that followed, Beryl notched up many other 'firsts': She was among the first in 1935 to help to successfully treat a child with streptococcal septicaemia using Prontosil, the fore-runner of the sulphonamides; she was one of the first to treat a baby with Rh haemolytic disease using Rh negative blood; that was in 1943; in 1945 she was one of the first women doctors to be elected to membership of the previously exclusively male Bristol Paediatric Association. In 1947 she was the first clinical lecturer in paediatrics in the South West Region. In the mid-1940s, she was the first paediatrician in England to set up a service for newborn babies, a subject to which I will return in a moment. In 1948 she was the first paediatrician in this country in over 100 years to successfully rear quadruplets: the Good quads.

She was one of the first, in 1949, to appreciate that premature infants might suffer brain damage from severe jaundice and to appreciate the need for exchange transfusion in order to prevent

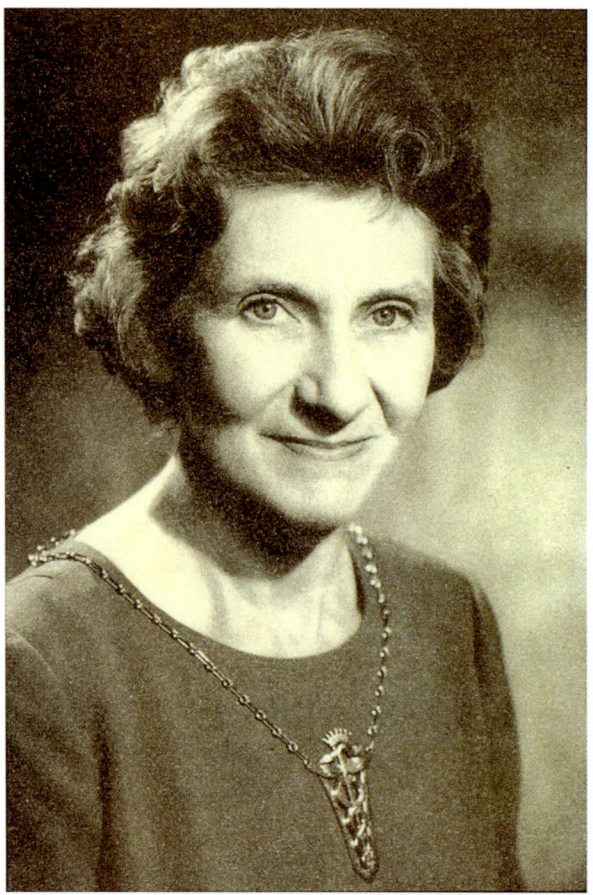

Fig 3 Dr. Beryl Corner, 1963

it. She was the first (and it has to be said, the last) to use methyl scopolamine in 1955 to treat pyloric stenosis medically.

With Bill Gillespie, in 1960, she was the first to demonstrate the value of hexachloraphane in banishing staphylococcal infection from our nurseries. Then with the MRC she was one of the team to first study the value of streptomycin in the treatment of TB meningitis and also to investigate the cause of blindness in premature infants due to excess of oxygen. It is not easy to estimate how many infant and child lives were saved by her initiatives and care.

It is still difficult to imagine Bristol without Beryl (Fig 3). She was, of course, a very small person, especially in later years. The sight of her huge white Mercedes moving in a stately fashion through the traffic without apparently having anyone at the wheel, struck fear into the heart of many a motorist. Nor were motorists the only ones to feel fear. When Beryl arrived on a ward round, even the most innocent experienced a peculiar sense of discomfort in case they had in some way done wrong. You have to appreciate that Beryl had been schooled in a chauvinistic male-dominated medical world. She had to be tough to survive – and survive she did in fine style although, to be honest, she was not always an easy colleague. Yet to her juniors, especially if they were women, she gave unstinted encouragement. Indeed she took a tremendous interest in, and care of, both medical students and young doctors-in-training coming from around the world, inspiring them with her dedication and talents, and providing them with friendly – and also sometimes financial – support when the need arose.

A few years ago, I asked Beryl what she considered to be her most important achievement. Without hesitation she replied: *'The establishment of newborn care as a paediatric responsibility'.* I wish she could be here to tell you the story herself because it is quite a story but if she were here, I have to tell you, you would probably miss your lunch!

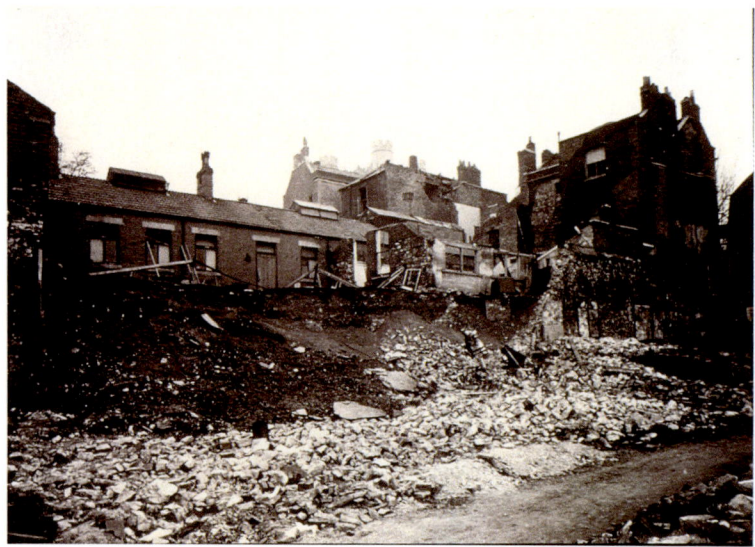

Fig 4 Bombing of the Bristol Children's Hospital in 1942

Instead I will mention just a few of the highlights: in 1942 at the height of the war when the Blitz was on and the Bristol Children's Hospital was bombed (Fig 4), Beryl and Matron had to re-enter the damaged hospital at night to recover a baby patient that had been left behind by mistake. At that time, Beryl was running virtually single-handed the whole paediatric service in Bristol. It was then that the Chief Medical Officer, Professor Parry, invited her to take on responsibility from the obstetricians for the care of all the newborn in the City. Without hesitation she accepted. Her first action was to visit Dr. Victoria Mary Crosse in Birmingham who had set up a service for premature babies at Sorrento Hospital in the 1930s, and to study her methods.

Back in Bristol, Beryl set about introducing a neonatal service from scratch with the most minimum resources. Doctors, midwives and nurses required training, neonatal records had to be designed and equipment purchased. In 1946 she opened at Southmead Hospital, with Sister Luffman, the first Special Care Baby Unit for newborn infants in the UK. In 1948 a breast milk bank, possibly the first in the country, was also opened there. At that time too, she introduced an out-reach premature baby team of health visitors, able to follow up these vulnerable babies after they had returned home. In 1966 Beryl designed a brand new SCBU at Southmead Hospital (Fig 5).

Her own special interest was in the neuro-developmental follow-up of small, premature babies. Eventually, in 1960, she published all her experience in a text book called 'Prematurity'. I remember it well as my consultant in Birmingham at that time gave it to me as a Christmas present.

Beryl's activities extended way beyond her clinical paediatric duties; among them one might mention air-raid medical duties, Red Cross work, lecturing and teaching, and even ministering to the animals of Bristol Zoo and especially to her beloved baby apes, eight of

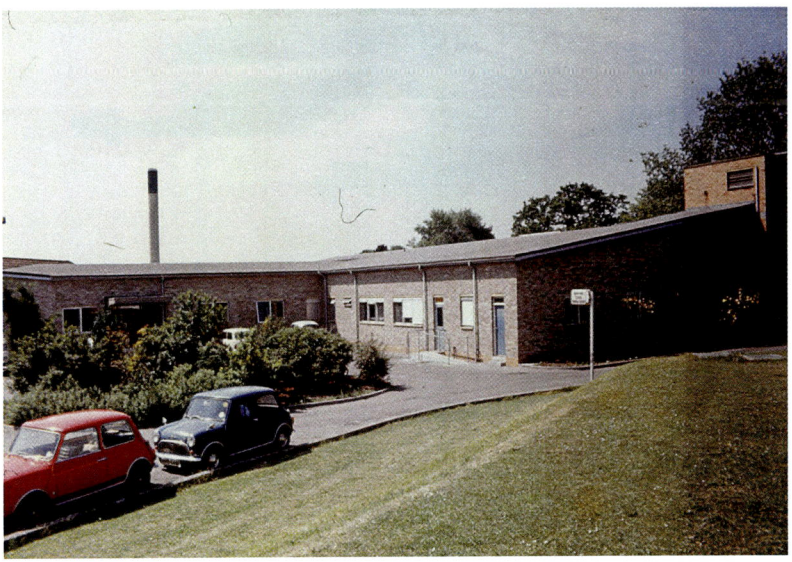

Fig 5 The Special Care Baby Unit, Southmead Hospital, opened 1966

which she cared for including one in the Special Care Unit of the old Bristol Maternity Hospital.

Apart from her many contributions in the UK, Beryl also undertook sterling work abroad, especially in India and the Far East, on behalf of the World Health Organisation and the British Council. Back in Bristol, there were duties as a magistrate and work for the Prison and Probation Services. She was also deeply involved with her old school, Redland High School for Girls, and in activities at Christchurch. A founder member of the Southmead Hospital orchestra, she was also director of the Bristol Music Club. Not for nothing, she was elected president of the Medical Women's International Association in 1978. This was one of at least eight presidencies that she undertook over the years, including: the paediatric section of the Royal Society of Medicine; the Society for the Study of In-born Errors of Metabolism; the Bristol Medico Churugical Society, the Bristol branch of the BMA; the South West Paediatric Club; the Women's Medical Federation; and, of course, the Bristol Medico-Historical Society. She was a founder member of the Neonatal Society and also an Honorary Fellow of the Royal College of Paediatrics and Child Health and of the British Association of Perinatal Medicine.

I should also mention that she gave the first Mary Crosse Memorial Lecture in 1976 following the death of her great friend, Vicki, some four years earlier. Also, in 2005, as the oldest Fellow present, she gave the Royal College of Physicians' vote of thanks to their President, Carol Black, on her remitting office. Beryl was 95 at the time. Her intellect remained as sharp as ever.

Beryl's achievements on behalf of children and in particular on behalf of the newborn did not go unnoticed. She was hailed both on television and in the press as a pioneer of newborn care in this country. In 1996 the University of Bristol awarded her the Degree of Doctor of Medicine, honoris causa, in recognition of her achievements. The University of the West of England also made her an Honorary Doctor of Science. In 2006 Beryl received an OBE from the hands of Prince Charles. Her nieces, Jane and Sally, who accompanied her to Buckingham Palace, have told me that it was a wonderful occasion and a fitting climax to a life devoted to the service of paediatrics and child health. It certainly gave Beryl the greatest pleasure. May she rest in peace. We, for our part, can only rejoice and give thanks for her truly remarkable life.'

Nutrition and the Death Camps

Stella Dilke
Presented March 2010

INTRODUCTION

Bergen-Belsen Concentration Camp was an institution originally established for prominent Jewish prisoners of the Third Reich (known as exchange Jews) but, by July 1944, had become a dumping ground for criminals, internees from other concentration camps of the Third Reich and political prisoners. Belsen was not an extermination camp like Auschwitz and prior to 1944 was considered to be one of the better camps, where Jews would work but "be kept healthy and alive"[1]. However, on arrival of the evacuees from the death camps of the East at the end of 1944, conditions within Belsen had become drastically overcrowded and thousands of internees in the camp were dying of starvation, typhus, typhoid fever and tuberculosis. By March 1945, 500-600 prisoners were dying each day and 1,000 inmates were visibly ill with typhus[2].

On liberation by the British on the 15th April 1945, Belsen was estimated to contain 60,000 people, most of whom were emaciated, lice ridden and apathetic due to starvation and of which 13,000 died post-liberation[3].

The relief effort at Bergen-Belsen is viewed in various lights historically. It is either extolled as a British triumph; that on discovery of 60,000 starving, infection-ridden prisoners of war, the British military had rallied London's medical schools, shipped in nutritional experts, moved prisoners out of Belsen into newly prepared, nearby hospital facilities to relatively swift recovery and as a final defiance of Nazism and burnt the most notorious part of Belsen, hoisting a Union Jack over it to symbolise a new beginning for the camp[4]. This version of the liberation cites the British as the saviours of the internees and is supported by the published accounts by both the military and medical staff present at the liberation of Belsen.

Naturally, to perpetuate this idea of the British within Belsen was advantageous to the British Government as anti-Fascist propaganda[5]. To be seen to uncover such evil had placed the British in a unique post-war position as Britain had fought from the very beginning against Nazism and was now responsible for the rehabilitation of its victims. It would garner worldwide respect.

The contrasting account to this paragon of goodness is the argument suggesting that although the British had known about the existence of concentration camps and the systematic destruction of the Jewish people for at least two years[6], and equally had known from the Germans on arrival that there were 60,000 internees in Belsen and an outbreak of typhus, they had not arrived prepared for the task at hand with no provisions for operations or most other medical interventions[7]. Equally, there is an argument which proposes the British had used the inmates of Belsen as guinea pigs to prepare for the relief of countries like Holland which were experiencing famine post-war.

My attempt to choose between these two contrasting accounts, to determine which the most accurate perception of the relief effort is, focuses on the medical interventions of the British, specifically in their treatment and actions regarding starvation within the camp addressing the problem of the dichotomy presented by historians at Belsen.

FEEDING THE 60,000

In May 1945, the military began tackling the colossal liberation task by evacuating internees out of Camp 1 into ad hoc hospitals whilst 97 London medical students who had been shipped in to aid in the relief effort[8] each commandeered a hut within Camp 19. The students attempted to distribute food and medical care and helped choose (via a form of triage) which patients would be taken to hospital for further care. After the evacuation of internees to these simple hospitals which were staffed with relatively fit internees (who acted as nurses), the United Nations Relief and Rehabilitation Administration (UNRAA), who spearheaded the international aid effort, provided senior nurses and established regular nursing routines and more advanced medical care within the camp.

The most immediate problem for the British Army when Belsen was liberated was the mass starvation among its inmates. Initially, on discovery of the nightmarish conditions within the camp – thousands of half naked, human skeletons wandering around and keeling over from starvation[10] - the British had handed out all the Army basic rations they had available to the internees; tinned stew, biscuits and cigarettes[11]. However, after noting the excessive diarrhoea and vomiting caused by this rich diet and subsequent death of many due to perforated small bowels, the liberators had to assess the diets to be administered[12].

The realisation that a highly calorific diet would not aid the survivors in recovery from starvation prompted the British to bring in a nutritional expert named Jack Drummond[13]. The Medical Research Council (MRC) equally sent in a team of scientists lead by Dr Janet Vaughan[14]. The Medical Research Council at the time was a well respected research organisation funded by the Government, thus their role in Belsen would be purely experimental[15].

Both teams had various therapies to administer to the internees in an attempt to revive them from starvation. The MRC team specifically would try out a form of artificial nutrition known as protein hydrolysate[16], and the diet recommended by Jack Drummond was the Bengal Famine Mixture[17].

The administration of protein hydrolysate (soluble milk proteins) given either intravenously, nasally or orally[18] was widely acknowledged as a disaster by both those involved in assessing the recovery of patients[19], and the patients themselves within Belsen[20]. Internees responded poorly to their taste, there was no notable improvement in recovery when compared to other treatments and the psychological effect of intravenous therapies after the cruelties inflicted by the SS within concentration camps meant that patients assumed that they were being killed or prepared for gas chambers on reception of these inoculations[21]. Despite prior success or supposed success of hydrolysates in treatment of starvation in Bengal, they were swiftly discontinued[22].

The protein hydrolysates had been administered by various teams to the internees. The medical students had been given instructive packs for their use and had attempted to give terminally starved patients hydrolysate within the huts that they were responsible for[23]. They had abandoned the treatment for practical reasons; many of the patients refused inoculation, disliked the taste of hydrolysate and had atrophied airways[24] thus forcing nasal tubes injured them. The chaotic method of food distribution within the huts and the difficulty of making sure that the chronically ill received food at all also meant efficacy of the treatment could not be established here.

Janet Vaughan's MRC scientists had set up a form of clinical trial which compared protein hydrolysate treatment with a skimmed milk version of the Bengal Famine mixture and with intravenous glucose serum mixture. The trial also confirmed that hydrolysates were not applicable within Belsen, both physiologically and psychologically. Vaughan's team picked subjects who were free from confounding diseases like typhus and only suffered from 'starvation disease' yet these patients did not improve when compared to the other test subjects[25] suffering acute anxiety throughout with some 'preferring to curl up and die rather than receive more'[26]. The trial had concluded that the skimmed milk diet was the most effective in the treatment of inanition and protein hydrolysate therapy was discontinued within the camp. Drummond stated that 'the failure of the F-treatment once again demonstrated the 'importance and significance of the psychological consequences of food shortage'[27].

The other scientific treatment for starvation tested at Belsen was the 'Bengal Famine mixture', a liquid diet developed by Jack Drummond in response to the Bengal Famine. This was delivered in two forms: either as a gruel composed of flour, molasses, salt and water[28] which was served with glucose solution and vitamin tablets or as a solution of skimmed milk, glucose, salt and vitamin tablets[29]. Reception of these diets at Belsen was mixed, especially of the flour based one, and indeed the accounts of those present at Belsen either regarded it as a miracle cure[30] or as a highly unsuccessful solution to the starvation problem[31]. However, it must be noted that many of the eyewitness accounts are very difficult to trust in their accuracy; some survivors published their accounts in later life, suggesting that details may have been forgotten or bolstered by later official accounts of what happened in Belsen and many of the authors of accounts published around the time of liberation were liberators, thus deeply patriotic[32]. So retrospective evaluation of the relief strategies are, at least in part, clouded by conflicting accounts.

The Rabbi at Belsen, Leslie Hardman suggested that patients found the Bengal Famine Mixture too sweet for their Eastern European tastes and that the addition of paprika to the mixture had made it palatable[33]. This evidence was also supported by Janet Vaughan who concluded that the that the skimmed milk version of the Bengal Famine mixture was the most effective in revival of the internees but only when infused with flavours that they knew, such as coffee or cocoa due to the psychological need of the patients to remember the joy of eating[34].

However, Hardman also asserts that the Bengal famine mixture was a failure as a treatment generally and that patients experienced digestive problems on ingestion which he discussed with Jack Drummond[35]. This claim is countered by evidence suggesting that patients hoarded all food made available to them[36], sometimes in highly unsanitary conditions and for days. Thus, rather than caused by Bengal Famine mixture, the persistent diarrhoea and vomiting experienced by many internees could be attributed to ingestion of the hoarded food, failed digestion by atrophied small bowels and the presence of opportunistic pathogens[37]. Indeed, Hardman himself became ill after sharing hoarded food as part of religious celebrations within the camp[38] and this hypothesis is supported by Captain Mollison at Belsen who lamented the frequent relapses of diarrhoea in internees in the Belsen hospital, caused by their friends sneaking them bilberries[39].

Thus, the action of Hardman, kindly handing out all the food available against medical procedure may have inadvertently caused some of the malady[40].

When UNRAA nurses arrived in Belsen (as the second tier of relief) they expressed dismay at the primitive hospital conditions established; patients were residing in filthy straw palliases with a hundred patients cared for by one trained medical professional and various untrained internees. The nurses set about setting up regular feeding routines for patients as opposed to general distribution of food, recruited local German nurses to aid in the hospitals and employed a system of human laundry; DDT spraying and showering were made mandatory to admission to the hospital.

Three diets for internees were used universally throughout the camp from this point. Internees were ranked on a scale dependent on their ability to move around the camp and contribute to the relief effort[41].

Muriel Knox Doherty, a senior nurse at Belsen noted that [40] tonnes of dried skimmed milk had been brought in for this protocol despite the internees' belief that this diet had caused their diarrhoea and vomiting[42]. We could make the assumption that the adoption of this skimmed milk protocol was a result of Janet Vaughan's clinical trial and indeed the graded three tiered skimmed milk diet had been tried and tested by Lipscomb at Belsen using various increases in calories for internees with the three scale diet illustrated above being the most successful[43]. Yet, the evidence asserted by Vaughan's team regarding the efficacy of the Bengal Famine Diet had already been asserted by Indian nutritionists during the Bengal famine, where the tiered diet was first developed and applied[44]. Thus, one can surmise that the actual purpose of Janet Vaughan's trial (besides testing the worth of hydrolysates) was nullified.

The MRC's strategies later became the focus for ethical debates over the importance and value of patient autonomy. But we must be cautious to judge these strategies retrospectively. It is worth noting that the value of patient autonomy at this point in time was not encoded in ethical conventions or practices. In other medical fields at this time, especially within psychiatry, patient autonomy was wholly disregarded and consent was not part of the medical status quo. Moreover, one can question the value of consent in the context of Belsen. If thousands of patients were apathetic and speechless with hunger, what good would consent have been? The key ethical questions regarding the trial, in my opinion, lie in the motive behind the clinical trial which I shall discuss later.

The high energy skimmed milk Bengal Famine diet was retained in Belsen and gradually internees began to recover. It equally was adopted in the liberation of other concentration camps around the newly deposed Third Reich[45].

This chronology of events must now be considered within the history of nutrition.

STARVATION AND WORLD WAR II

World War II is widely considered to be the first war in which governmental forces worldwide began to realise the importance of good nutrition and an understanding of the science of nutrition, within both the armed forces and in the civilian population[46]. This revolution in food awareness had occurred after biochemists like Jack Drummond assessed exactly how many calories were required per day per individual[47] and had been successful in isolating vital vitamins such as vitamin A[48] and, after the military had realised that diseases such as typhus (or famine fever) were associated with poor nutrition[49] and that epidemics of measles were promptly followed by episodes of kwashiorkor[50]. This new found connection between war time disease and quality of nutrition was a justification for investment in appropriate food for the armed forces.

The importance and benefits of appropriate wartime nutrition were also applied to the general population. With food shortages and blockades between Britain and Europe, the calorific nature of food and the amount deemed necessary per person was vital for knowing the amount of food to ration optimally without endangering food stocks. Numerous historical and epidemiological studies have shown that the effects of science based rationing during and after the war had a positive effect on the overall health of the nation[51], and the general health of Britain's population was deemed to be better post war than before[52].

Yet, despite the increased drive to understand the sciences of nutrition, the scientific understanding of starvation and famine medicine during the Second World War was still underdeveloped when compared with the complex famine and relief related medical knowledge available today.

In 1942, A.C. Ivy in the United States had carried out tests with Dexedrine and caffeine to learn about physical endurance and weight loss[53]. In the Warsaw Ghetto between

1940 and 1942; starving polish doctors had recorded the effects of starvation in a still widely used set of papers which collaboratively are published under the title Hunger Disease[54]. This set of studies, published in 1946 from surviving doctors in the trial significantly stressed the importance of carbohydrate metabolism within starvation[55] a conclusion universally reached by the rest of the scientific community on publication of papers refuting the importance of protein in the treatment of inanition[56], and also noted by recovering doctors in communist prisoner of war camps in 1947[57].

In Bengal (during the famine of 1942-1943), Indian Doctors had published studies concerning the symptoms of hunger disease[58] and nutritionist Jack Drummond and Indian physicians Krishan, Narayanan and Sankaran had developed treatments for the starving based on their physiology. Yet, despite worldwide scientific endeavour 'the glaring omissions indicated that what one arm of Allied intelligence knew was not divulged to the other.'[59] The wartime disruption of the global scientific community meant that pieces of correlating information– from Warsaw, the United States, from Communist Russia etc. could not be collaborated until after the war, thus would have had little relevance to the work within Belsen, aside from the research supplied from the Bengal Famine by Jack Drummond and by Krishan et al which was promoted by the MRC[60].

The Bengal Famine took place between 1943 and 1944 and was widely considered to have occurred because of a minimal increase in the price of rice[61] resulting in the starvation of millions of Indian farmers[62]. The famine was very severe and resulted in millions of Indian deaths. Despite the relative anonymity of the Bengal Famine in contrast to the other events occurring between 1942 and 1943, the observations of famine from India provided the scientific community with a good idea of the physiology of starvation; papers published in the BMJ and Lancet examined the onset of famine oedema and the lack of vitamin deficiency in full blown emaciation, citing the papers from India as evidence[63]. Yet, among British researchers, the famine gained new significance in the context of starvation work in the death camps. Thus, the bulk of discussion regarding the Bengal Famine was published after the British first entered Belsen (the British entered in April, starvation publications from Bengal appeared predominantly in June 1945). It would appear however, that protein hydrolysates had the least evidence supporting their use from Bengal.

Medical interest in Protein hydrolysates had begun in 1913 when Henriques and Anderson injected goats with pancreatic extract of goat flesh and noted nitrogen equilibrium[64], but they were only practically applied medically in 1938 by Elman and Weiner[65]. They were used experimentally in 1942[66] but were only deployed on a larger scale in the treatment of the 'sick starving destitutes'[67] in Bengal.

Three Indian doctors (Krishan et al) had experimented with hydrolysates in Calcutta in the form of injected extract of papain[68] which they had shown to yield positive results[69] in the treatment of inanition.[70] The limited experimental evidence from this trial suggested that hydrolysate reduced the death rate from starvation by 50%[71].

After the trial, the Indian government allowed the treatment to be utilised as a treatment of starvation among the starving Bengali population with vague measurement of its effect. The reaction of the Indian press to the use of protein hydrolysate treatment however, was highly critical. The press hypothesized that the 'F' Treatment[72] had no practical application and that its use was only political; to prevent the vilification of the civil services who had reacted badly to the famine and provided ineffectual relief far too late. Equally, it had been suggested that the starving in India were being used as guinea pigs for this controversial 'F' treatment[73].

From a purely scientific basis, the experimental evidence for the efficacy of hydrolysate was not supported by good enough evidence in the initial papers or by further trials with proven efficacy, especially when compared with other therapies at the time (like the fluid Bengal diets). The efficacy of hydrolysate was highly debated within the scientific community in India alone, let alone within the global scientific community and the less organised testing of the treatment within the Bengal Famine had yielded mixed results.

Protein hydrolysate continued to be tested for at least ten years after the Bengal Famine, yielding extremely positive results when conventional trial methods were employed[74]. However, there was still little support for the use of hydrolysate in Belsen other than the initial papers, therefore its employment at Belsen was highly experimental and not fully justified.

Unlike hydrolysate, the use of the Bengal Famine Diet within Belsen appears to be completely legitimate. Jack Drummond had developed the Bengal Famine Mixture after being sent in to deal with the crisis in Bengal and it had garnered some success in India[75]. The diet formulated had the same two forms used as in Belsen: a skimmed milk version (with added eggs and shark liver oil[76]) and a flour based version with similar extra ingredients. Drummond's diet had been employed by the Indian government to be administered under strict protocol to the starving[77] and British Medical Officers had followed the protocol of the tiered diet in Bengal and had relayed information regarding its efficacy to Belsen[78].

Despite some criticism by military doctors of the diet[79], the skimmed milk version was also utilised in the liberation of Sandbostel[80] and in various Japanese prisoner of war camps[81]. And, after the WHO renamed the skimmed milk Bengal Famine mixture to 'The high energy milk diet'[82], it continued to be used following the three tiered system pioneered in India.

We can therefore assert that Jack Drummond pioneered a treatment in Bengal that is still medically relevant in the treatment of starvation[83] and that the British use of the Bengal Famine mixture was justified in its prescription to reanimate the internees of Belsen, but that the use of the protein hydrolysates had less justification for use, except as a final resort for those who could not orally ingest food.

MOTIVES AND DICHOTOMIES

The Belsen Clinical Trial, conducted by Janet Vaughan and her team of MRC scientists was requested by L.T. Poole, Director of Pathology for the War Office[84] in the three week gap between the discovery of Belsen and the initiation of the Bengal based therapies. Poole, an Army Captain and pathologist had been responsible for the utilisation of penicillin within Second World War[85] and had published various articles discussing its efficacy and use within the army[86]. Penicillin had been one of the flagship medicines pioneered within World War II and a lasting rivalry between Axis and Allied medical research had existed throughout the war.[87]

The utilisation of these new medicines within World War II had been greatly successful for the British; penicillin had saved many lives, the use of DDT against typhus had prevented frontline epidemics from occurring and had proved useful in the disinfection of populations[88]. Experiments conducted by characters like Poole on gangrene and wounds had resulted in efficient and relatively healthy troops throughout[89].

The fact that Poole (who was at the frontline of wartime medical experimentation in Britain) was responsible for the decision to initiate the Belsen hydrolysate trial suggests that the repercussions of experiments proving that protein hydrolysate was successful in revival of the starving would have been many fold. Hugh Stannus suggested around that time that hydrolysates 'had sprung rather suddenly into prominence, and might attain the unenviable position of being regarded as a cure for all'[90,91]

The effects of hydrolysate treatment on the future of military and starvation medicine, if it were successful, were not exaggerated. By 1945, the possibility of PoW camps containing starving British troops across the world was a serious one. If hydrolysate worked as a treatment, these soldiers could be fed quickly and brought back to the front line. Equally, as hydrolysates were relatively simple to produce and utilise, frontline medical care within military medicine would be revolutionised; soldiers could carry emergency supplies and military doctors could carry around substantial stocks for utilisation when necessary[92].

Practically, the internees were a useful population for experimentation. Of the 60,000 people contained within the camp, most internees had no individual records or any information regarding their status as citizens within their home countries, as most had been destroyed on entrance to any of the German concentration camps[93] and, any notable internees had been shipped out of Belsen as soon as the liberation took place[94].

Following this, this would surely be an ideal population for experimentation. This appears to be asserted by the use of Belsen internees for vascular injury trials by British scientists who were requested to join Janet Vaughan at Belsen 'to carry out (as much[95]) research as possible'[96].

Equally, the British had had awareness of the systematic removal of Jews from European countries[97] and had constant relief requests from Jewish groups within Great Britain to send aid to concentration camps. These requests had been refused by the British government to prevent an impression of favouritism towards a particular minority group, both from a domestic and international viewpoint[98]. This refusal to give aid before liberation and the continued bombing of concentration camps by the British Government does not particularly support the claim that the British cared about the fate of the Jews within the Third Reich.

Despite the presence of journalists like Richard Dimbleby who had been present at the liberation and had made their opinions regarding the matter widely known, and the widespread knowledge of the existence of Belsen post liberation, the British government had full control over the press and publication of the actions of the liberators. The clinical trial was a guarded secret with documents regarding it marked as 'confidential' and of which details were only released for publication relatively recently[99]. Aside from controversies that 'arose in parts of the press about the effectiveness of the 'treatment' adopted by the team at Belsen, and its later application to the starving prisoners returning from Japanese camps'[100], the testing was kept clandestine and is not to be found in accounts published by the liberators, even that of Derrick Sington[101], thereby suggesting perhaps that military personnel were kept in the dark regarding the trial.

Regarding the motives for the trial, aside from idealistic estimations of the power of hydrolysates, Janet Vaughan's friends state that she went to Belsen to investigate the efficacy of hydrolysate in order for the British to develop starvation relief to send to the Dutch to aid with their famine[102] and that Belsen was the perfect opportunity to do this. The other account states that the MRC team was diverted from Holland where they had been initially sent, to Belsen with large stocks of hydrolysate in order to respond to the emergency. There are several problems with both of these accounts.

Firstly, the Dutch famine had been going on for two years and both the Red Cross and the British government had sent aid from the beginning of 1945[103]. Secondly, by April 1945 the serious effects of the Dutch famine had started to wane, and the Dutch had started to recover. Hydrolysates would be inappropriate within this setting as the Dutch still had a sizeable working population, who although they would require extra calorific intake would not be so emaciated as to require hydrolysate to the degree specified in Bengal. Equally, as quoted previously, hydrolysate was also utilised in the liberation of Japanese prisoner of war camps which would have contained British soldiers.

The excuse of sending aid to the Dutch had also been employed with the Belsen medical students, who had arrived at Belsen expecting to be sent to Holland to help there. If the British were not fully aware of the extent of relief required in

Holland then the first excuse: that 'three weeks before teams of British Nutritionists were dispatched to the Netherlands, an unexpected opportunity arose to test the efficacy of the F-Treatment when Belsen was liberated'[104] can be deemed the most plausible for the direct requirement for testing of hydrolysate.

The motives illustrated above do not present a particularly favourable impression of the British government, but I think the main point to emphasise is that of the motive of the British War Office and not that of the military, of whom as mentioned, had doctors who objected to the trials within Belsen. As suggested motive for the trial, it appears likely that the War Office had exploited the Belsen internees in order to aid their own troops in the Middle East, but the potential repercussions of hydrolysate treatment for the internees if proven successful and the presence of Jack Drummond had been in the best interest of the internees.

CONCLUSION

When examining a historical case a complicated as this, with arguably three parties involved (the military, the War Office and UNRAA), it would appear that the dichotomy of the liberation lies within the actions of these three groups. The reaction of the world to the action of the military personnel responsible for liberation was relatively favourable[105]. The work of the UNRAA nurses in Belsen, more so[106]. This can be contrasted with the secretive and unethical nature of the clinical trial controlled by the British War Office. The contrast of these three groups and their involvement in the liberation refutes any possibility of deeming the actions of the British as either good or bad, and questions the arguments of historians like Paul Weindling and Joanne Reilly in their dichotomised views of the liberation. From a nutritional standpoint alone, the British are shown to behave in both exemplary and despicable fashions.

It is equally difficult to question the ethics of the medical and military staff at Belsen by modern standards, as the protocol of clinical equipoise and the importance of patient autonomy had not fully been established by this point. The actions and motives of the trial suggest that it did not take place wholly altruistically, but the results of the trial did have useful consequences, for both internees and future relief, as can been seen in the prolonged use of Vaughan's flavoured mixtures in disaster protocols[107], and in the use of Drummond's Famine Mixture by the WHO[108].

The liberation effort shows complex connections between political motive, military force and scientific endeavour, spelling the beginning of a new era in warfare- that is still highly relevant today. The interactions between these three forces, although united nationally, may provide a useful retrospective assessment of the worth of military science during and after the war. It may also indicate the benefit of the liberation to British government, instead of merely as a costly, lengthy and horrific procedure, as the therapies developed in Belsen proved to be very useful in the long term.

The liberation of Bergen-Belsen, as the first large camp of its kind to be liberated in the Third Reich, set a precedent regarding appropriate ways to rehabilitate the starving post war. It was a keystone event in history that simultaneously proved to the scientific community the importance of famine physiology during War and of the imperative to save further men around the world from dying of terminal starvation in this way. The Belsen legacy has great significance in the field of famine relief.

REFERENCES AND NOTES

1 Pg 12, as quoted by Heinrich Himmler on establishment of Belsen, Ben Shephard, After Daybreak, The Liberation of Bergen-Belsen 1945. 1st Edn. (United States: Schocken Books 2005)
2 Pg 21, Ben Shephard, After Daybreak, The Liberation of Bergen-Belsen 1945. 1st Edn. (United States: Schocken Books 2005)
3 ...either of terminal starvation or famine related diseases. Bergen-Belsen Memorial, Bergen-Belsen
4 Ibid.
5 Joanne Reilly, Belsen: The Liberation of a Concentration Camp, 1st Edn. (London: Routledge 1998)
6 Pg 827, Ronald W. Zweig, 'Feeding the Camps: Allied Blockade Policy and the relief of concentration camps in Germany 1944-1945', The Historical Journal, Vol. 41, No. 3, September 1998, pp 825-851
7 Pg 4, Ben Shepherd, After Daybreak, The Liberation of Bergen-Belsen 1945. 1st Edn. (United States: Schocken Books 2005)
8 Paul Kemp for the Imperial War Museum, The Relief of Belsen April 1945: Eyewitness Accounts. 1st Edn. (England: George Ove Ltd. 1991)
9 The original concentration camp
10 Pg 33, Derrick Sington, Belsen Uncovered, 1st Edn. (London: Duckworth Books 1946)
11 Ibid.
12 'The liberators had meant so well in giving us these generous rations, but had no experience of dealing with such starvation. How could they guess that the excellent food and generous quantities might have such a disastrous effect on starving people?'
Pg 62, Elisabeth Sommer-Lefkovis, Are you here in this hell too? Memories of troubled times 1944-1945, 1st Edn. (Oxford: Menard Press 1995). pg 62.
13 One of the most eminent nutritionists of the era and indeed perhaps in the history of nutritional science; Pg 49, Leslie H. Hardman, The Survivors, the story of the Belsen Remnant. 1st Edn. (London: Mitchell and Co. Ltd 1958)
14 .. a well respected haematologist from Oxford. Edited by Pauline Adams, Janet Maria Vaughan 1899-1993 A Memorial Tribute. (Oxford: Somerville College 1994)

15 They had pioneered the use of radiotherapy in the treatment of cancer and had been at the forefront of development of vaccines in the 1940's. MRC website: http://www.mrc.ac.uk/Achievementsimpact/Clinicaltrials/TheMRCandclinicaltrials/index.htm

16 E. Trepman, 'Rescue of the Remnants: The British Emergency Medical Relief Operation in Belsen Camp 1945', J R Army Med Corps 2001; 147: 281-293

17 ...which had been successful in treatment of the starving in Bengal, India in 1944 W.K. Aykroyd, The Conquest of Famine, 1st Edn. (London: Chatto and Windus 1974)

18 'Instructions for Use of Protein Hydrolysates', issued by the N.M.A. photocopied by Ben Shephard from the Wellcome Trust.

19 C.E. Dent, Rosalind Pitt Rivers and Janet Vaughan, 'Report of the comparative value of Hydrolysates, Milk and Serum in the treatment of starvation, based on observations made at Belsen Camp', Confidential Report commissioned by the Medical Research Council. Circulated 24th August 1945 to all members of the committee and 6 copies to Dr Vaughan. The National Archives. FD1/6346

20 Pg 17-18, Account of John Dixey, Medical Student at St Barts; Paul Kemp for the Imperial War Museum, The Relief of Belsen April 1945: Eyewitness Accounts. 1st Edn. (England: George Ove Ltd. 1991)

21 C.E. Dent, Rosalind Pitt Rivers and Janet Vaughan, 'Report of the comparative value of Hydrolysates, Milk and Serum in the treatment of starvation, based on observations made at Belsen

22 K.V.Krishan, K. Narayanan and G. Sankaran, 'Protein Hydrolysates in the treatment of Inanition', The Indian Medical Gazette, Vol 179 April 1944

23 'Instructions for Use of Protein Hydrolysates', issued by the N.M.A. photocopied by Ben Shephard from the Wellcome Trust.

24 Pg 18: letter from Alan MacAuslan, medical student at St Thomas's 'We tried to pass a nasal tube on her, to give her protein hydrolysate, but her nose was so atrophied and blocked, that we could not get the thin tube down, and part of the nasal conchae came adrift on the end of it.'
Paul Kemp for the Imperial War Museum, The Relief of Belsen April 1945: Eyewitness Accounts. 1st Edn. (England: George Ove Ltd. 1991)

25 C.E. Dent, Rosalind Pitt Rivers and Janet Vaughan, 'Report of the comparative value of Hydrolysates, Milk and Serum in the treatment of starvation, based on observations made at Belsen Camp', Confidential Report commissioned by the Medical Research Council. Circulated 24th August 1945 to all members of the committee and 6 copies to Dr Vaughan. The National Archives. FD1/6346

26 'Physiology and The Treatment of Starvation', BMJ, June 9th 1945

27 Pg 151, James Vernon, Hunger: A Modern History, (USA: Harvard University Press 2007)

28 Pg 49, Muriel Knox Doherty, Letters from Belsen 1945. 2nd Edn 2000 (Australia: Allen and Umain 2000)
29 Pg 78, All-Indian Institute of Hygiene and Public Health, 'Treatment and management of starving sick and destitute', The Indian Medical Gazette, February 1944 pp 73-81
30 Pg 63, Elisabeth Sommer-Lefkovis, Are you here in this hell too? Memories of troubled times 1944-1945, 1st Edn. (Oxford: Menard Press 1995).
31 Pg 49, Leslie H. Hardman, The Survivors, the story of the Belsen Remnant. 1st Edn. (London: Mitchell and Co. Ltd 1958)
32 Like Derrick Sington for example
33 Pg 49, Leslie H. Hardman, The Survivors, the story of the Belsen Remnant. 1st Edn. (London: Mitchell and Co. Ltd 1958)
34 C.E. Dent, Rosalind Pitt Rivers and Janet Vaughan, 'Report of the comparative value of Hydrolysates, Milk and Serum in the treatment of starvation, based on observations made at Belsen Camp', Confidential Report commissioned by the Medical Research Council. Circulated 24th August 1945 to all members of the committee and 6 copies to Dr Vaughan. The National Archives. FD1/6346
35 Pg 49, Leslie H. Hardman, The Survivors, the story of the Belsen Remnant. 1st Edn. (London: Mitchell and Co. Ltd 1958)
36 Pg 17: Major Hilda Roberts and Captain Petronella Potter, Paul Kemp for the Imperial War Museum, The Relief of Belsen April 1945: Eyewitness Accounts. 1st Edn. (England: George Ove Ltd. 1991)
37 Pg 18, Paul Kemp for the Imperial War Museum, The Relief of Belsen April 1945: Eyewitness Accounts. 1st Edn. (England: George Ove Ltd. 1991)
38 Pg 30, Leslie H. Hardman, The Survivors, the story of the Belsen Remnant. 1st Edn. (London: Mitchell and Co. Ltd 1958)
39 Pg 1, Report by Captain J.A. Mollison, 'Starvation in Belsen', War Office Report, National Archives, photocopied by Ben Shephard.
40 'I ignored the official order that 'No officer or other ranks must give the people additional food'. I felt, rightly or wrongly, that it was issued because of the army's inability to obtain more food, and not because of any injurious effect extra food might have.'
Pg 50, Leslie H. Hardman, The Survivors, the story of the Belsen Remnant. 1st Edn. (London: Mitchell and Co. Ltd 1958)
41 Scale No. 1: (Two hourly feeds for starved internees): Skimmed fresh or dried milk (2l) sugar (1oz) salt(1/2oz), compound vitamin tablets (3)
Scale No. 2: (diet for those not in hospital): compound above, bread, potatoes, flour, soup, tinned meat and veg.
Scale No. 3: (normal hospital diet): compound above but 1 1/2litre of milk, bread, potatoes, margarine, soup, tinned meat and veg41

Pg 49, Muriel Knox Doherty Letters from Belsen 1945. 2nd Edn 2000 (Australia: Allen and Umain 2000)
42 Pg 49, Muriel Knox Doherty Letters from Belsen 1945. 2nd Edn 2000 (Australia: Allen and Umain 2000)
43 Pg 503, R.O. Murray, 'Recovery from Starvation', The Lancet, April 19 1947
44 All-Indian Institute of Hygiene and Public Health, 'Treatment and management of starving sick and destitute', The Indian Medical Gazette, February 1944 pp 73-81
45 Clifford Barnard, Two weeks in May 1945 (London: Quaker Home Service 1999)
46 Mark Harrison, Medicine and Victory, British Military Medicine in the Second World War. (New York: Oxford University Press 2004)
47 Edited by Robert I. Rotberg and Theodore K. Rabb, Hunger and History: the impact of changing food production and consumption patterns on society, 1st Edn. (Cambridge: Cambridge University Press 1985)
48 Wikipedia entry: Jack Drummond
49 'The Conquest of Typhus' New York Times, 1944, National Library of Medicine
50 Pg 289, Edited by Robert I. Rotberg and Theodore K. Rabb, Hunger and History: the impact of changing food production and consumption patterns on society, 1st Edn. (Cambridge: Cambridge University Press 1985)
51 James Vernon, Hunger: A Modern History, (USA: Harvard University Press 2007)
52 Edited by Robert I. Rotberg and Theodore K. Rabb, Hunger and History: the impact of changing food production and consumption patterns on society, 1st Edn. (Cambridge: Cambridge University Press 1985)
53 Pg 24, Paul Julian Weindling, Nazi Medicine and the Nuremberg Trials, 1st Edn (Great Britain: Palgrave Macmillan Books 2004)
54 Edited by Myron Winick, Hunger Disease; studies by the Jewish Physicians in the Warsaw Ghetto, 2nd Edn (originally published 1946). (Canada: John Wileya Sons Ltd 1979)
55 Ibid.
56 Donald S. McLaren, 'The Great Protein Fiasco', The Lancet, July 13 1974
57 R.O. Murray, 'Recovery from Starvation', The Lancet, April 19 1947
58 K.S. Fitch, A Medical History of the Bengal Famine, (Calcutta: South of India Press 1947)
59 Pg 36, Pg 24, Paul Julian Weindling, Nazi Medicine and the Nuremberg Trials, 1st Edn (Great Britain: Palgrave Macmillan Books 2004)
60 C.E. Dent, Rosalind Pitt Rivers and Janet Vaughan, 'Report of the comparative value of Hydrolysates, Milk and Serum in the treatment of starvation, based on

observations made at Belsen Camp', Confidential Report commissioned by the Medical Research Council. Circulated 24th August 1945 to all members of the committee and 6 copies to Dr Vaughan. The National Archives. FD1/6346

61 www.prima.net/bowbrick/Cfam97/Bengal.htm 'How Sen's theory can cause famines'

62 Pg 731, 'Famine in Bengal', The Lancet, June 9th 1945 pp 731-732

63 'Physiology and The Treatment of Starvation', BMJ, June 9th 1945

64 Reports of Societies, 'Physiology and treatment of Starvation', BMJ, June 9 1945

65 Pg 237, Dr. A. B. Anderson (Glasgow Royal Infirmary), 'The Therapeutic Use of Protein Hydrolysates', Proceedings of the Nutrition Society (1946), Cambridge University Press

66 Pg 238, Dr. A. B. Anderson (Glasgow Royal Infirmary), 'The Therapeutic Use of Protein Hydrolysates', Proceedings of the Nutrition Society (1946), Cambridge University Press

67 All-Indian Institute of Hygiene and Public Health, 'Treatment and management of starving sick and destitute', The Indian Medical Gazette, February 1944 pp 73-81

68 K.V.Krishan, K. Narayanan and G. Sankaran, 'Protein Hydrolysates in the treatment of Inanition', The Indian Medical Gazette, Vol 179 April 1944

69 Pg 15, K.S. Fitch, A Medical History of the Bengal Famine, (Calcutta: South of India Press 1947)

70 to 'help to revive the cases quickly and enable them to take suitable diet by the mouth Pg 78, All-Indian Institute of Hygiene and Public Health, 'Treatment and management of starving sick and destitute', The Indian Medical Gazette, February 1944 pp 73-81

71 Pg 178, James Vernon, Hunger: A Modern History, (USA: Harvard University Press 2007)

72 The original name of protein hydrolysate treatment

73 'F Treatment' was the name of Protein Hydrolysate treatment developed in India.

Pg 148, James Vernon, Hunger: A Modern History, (USA: Harvard University Press 2007)

74 Fritz Lidström, 'Clinical and Experimental Studies on Intravenous Nutrition with a Dialyzed Enzymatic Casein Hydrolysate', Acta Chirurgica Scandinavica, (Stockholm: Kungl. Boktryckeriet P.A. Norstedt & Soner) Vol. 107 1954

75 K.S. Fitch, A Medical History of the Bengal Famine, (Calcutta: South of India Press 1947)

76 Pg 78, All-Indian Institute of Hygiene and Public Health, 'Treatment and management of starving sick and destitute', The Indian Medical Gazette,

February 1944
77 Ibid.
78 Pg 268, Mark Harrison, Medicine and Victory, British Military Medicine in the Second World War. (New York: Oxford University Press 2004)
79 Ibid.
80 Clifford Barnard, Two weeks in May 1945 (London: Quaker Home Service 1999)
81 Janet Maria Vaughan 1899-1993 A Memorial Tribute. (Oxford: Somerville College 1994)
82 Lindsay H. Allen, 'Interventions for Micronutrient Deficiency Control in Developing Countries: Past, Present and Future', The American Society for Nutritional Sciences, November 2003
83 C.E. Dent, Rosalind Pitt Rivers and Janet Vaughan, 'Report of the comparative value of Hydrolysates, Milk and Serum in the treatment of starvation, based on observations made at Belsen Camp', Confidential Report commissioned by the Medical Research Council. Circulated 24th August 1945 to all members of the committee and 6 copies to Dr Vaughan. The National Archives. FD1/6346
84 C.E. Dent, Rosalind Pitt Rivers and Janet Vaughan, 'Report of the comparative value of Hydrolysates, Milk and Serum in the treatment of starvation, based on observations made at Belsen Camp', Confidential Report commissioned by the Medical Research Council. Circulated 24th August 1945 to all members of the committee and 6 copies to Dr Vaughan. The National Archives. FD1/6346
85 Pg 303, H.W.Florey, E.P. Abraham, 'The Work on Penicillin at Oxford', http://jhmas.oxfordjournals.org/cgi/reprint/VI/Summer/302.pdf
86 .. a spray pump had been developed to allow women to retain their modesty and still killed typhus ridden lice effectively. L.T. Poole, 'British Progress with Penicillin', British Journal of Surgery, No. 32, 1944
87 H.W.Florey, E.P. Abraham, 'The Work on Penicillin at Oxford'
88 'The Conquest of Typhus' New York Times, 1944, National Library of Medicine
89 L.T. Poole, 'Review of the Florey and Cairns Report on the Use of Penicillin in War Wounds', Journal of Neurosurgery, May 1944, Vol. 1, No. 3, Pages 201-210
90 'Physiology and The Treatment of Starvation', BMJ, June 9th 1945
91 This is echoed by characters like Richard Magee in the United States, who had expressed his belief in the pleuripotent nature of hydrolysate in the treatment of the starving, noting the stockpile of hydrolysate by the Ministry of Health for immediate use.
Ibid.
92 'Instructions for Use of Protein Hydrolysates', issued by the N.M.A.

photocopied by Ben Shephard from the Wellcome Trust.

93'It became apparent early in April, 1945, that the advancing armies in Europe might be expected to liberate large numbers of people suffering from severe starvation. Uncontrolled clinical observations made at the time of the Bengal famine (Krishnan and Narayanan, 1944) suggested that such people would be unable to take food by mouth and that intravenous therapy with protein hydrolysates was far more effective than treatment with plasma transfusion. It was imperative therefore, to determine by controlled clinical and biochemical observations how far oral and intravenous hydrolysate might be effective in the treatment of severe starvation in Europeans'93.

Edited by Jo Reilly, David Cesarani, Tony Kushner, Colin Richmond, Belsen in History & Memory, 1st Edn. (Great Britain: Frank Cass and Co Ltd. 1997)

94 Ronald W. Zweig, 'Feeding the Camps: Allied Blockade Policy and the relief of concentration camps in Germany 1944-1945', The Historical Journal, Vol. 41, No. 3, September 1998, pp 825-851

95 My addition, in context of the article.

96 Pg 1,Report by Captain J.A. Mollison, 'Starvation in Belsen', WO, National Archives

97 Edited by Suzanne Bardgett and David Cesarani, 'Special Issue, Belsen 1945, New Historical Perspectives', Holocaust Studies, a Journal of Culture and History, Volume 12 Summer/Autumn 2006 Numbers 1-2

98 Ronald W. Zweig, 'Feeding the Camps: Allied Blockade Policy and the relief of concentration camps in Germany 1944-1945', The Historical Journal, Vol. 41, No. 3, September 1998

99 C.E. Dent, Rosalind Pitt Rivers and Janet Vaughan, 'Report of the comparative value of Hydrolysates, Milk and Serum in the treatment of starvation, based on observations made at Belsen Camp', Confidential Report commissioned by the Medical Research Council. Circulated 24th August 1945 to all members of the committee and 6 copies to Dr Vaughan. The National Archives. FD1/6346

100 Edited by Pauline Adams, Janet Maria Vaughan 1899-1993 A Memorial Tribute. (Oxford: Somerville College 1994)

101 who was a journalist prior to entering the army

102 Edited by Pauline Adams, Janet Maria Vaughan 1899-1993 A Memorial Tribute. (Oxford: Somerville College 1994)

103 Nicky Hart, 'Famine, maternal nutrition and infant mortality: a re-examination of the Dutch Hunger Winter, population studies, Vol. 47, No. 1, March 1993 pp27-46

104 Ronald W. Zweig, 'Feeding the Camps: Allied Blockade Policy and the relief of concentration camps in Germany 1944-1945', The Historical Journal, Vol.

41, No. 3, September 1998, pp 825-851
105 Pg 18, Paul Kemp for the Imperial War Museum, The Relief of Belsen April 1945: Eyewitness Accounts. 1st Edn. (England: George Ove Ltd. 1991)
106 Pg 80, Leslie H. Hardman, The Survivors, the story of the Belsen Remnant. 1st Edn. (London: Mitchell and Co. Ltd 1958)
107 Pg 85, 'Famine, a symposium dealing with Nutrition and Relief Operations in Times of Disaster', Symposia of the Swedish Nutrition Foundation 1X. (Sweden: Almquist and Wikselis Uppsala 1971)
108 Pg 87, 'Famine, a symposium dealing with Nutrition and Relief Operations in Times of Disaster', Symposia of the Swedish Nutrition Foundation 1X. (Sweden: Almquist and Wikselis Uppsala 1971)

Medical Aspects of the Younghusband Mission to Tibet

Vincent Marmion

Emeritus Consultant, Bristol Eye Hospital

Presented 17.9.2012

The Young husband Mission to Tibet came to my attention as the third house surgeon trained at the Bristol Eye Hospital (1895-7), Thomas Bernard Kelly, was an Indian Medical Service surgeon who endured the full ten months it took to complete the mission entrusted to Colonel Francis Younghusband CFY. The latter by chance had been a pupil at Clifton College. Francis Younghusband was commissioned by the Viceroy Lord Curzon to reach an agreement with the Tibetan authorities, essentially the Dali Lama, on a taxation issue. This arose as the Tibetans had, over a long period, levied taxes on goods in transit from China, Tibet was under Chinese rule and the taxes had already been paid to the Chinese authorities. It appears there was no justification for this additional tax.

Over a frustrating six months Younghusband attempted to reach an agreement with the Tibetan authorities who constantly prevaricated and on Lord Curzon's instructions an escorted mission was raised. They set out in early December 1903. Their primary objective was to reach Guyantse, the second town in Tibet and establish a base there by January. There they were to negotiate with the Tibetan representatives. The movement of a party which was about one thousand strong up the luscious Teesta Valley to Pari Jong on the border with Tibet. This was beset with major problems amongst the pack animals. From Langram, two thousand feet below the Jalap La pass (at 12,000 ft), the track was basically a series of 'stairs'.

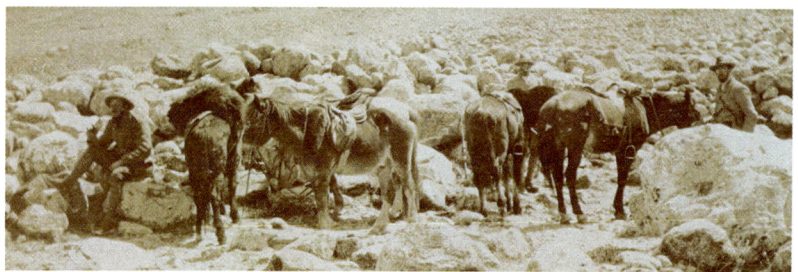

*Figure 1: Lt MacLeod Captains R Fearon and T B Kelly March 1904
Photo 1083/13/ 75 &6 reproduced with the kind permission of the British Library.*

The majority of supplies and baggage had to be carried by porters and much less on mules.

Once over the pass into Tibet they were in the wooded Chumbi Valley the first village was Gnatong. The hovels there were so unsatisfactory that they moved further on to Dotha (figure 1) where they pitched tents and there they celebrated Christmas. At the end of the month they surmounted the Tang La pass and on the 8th January reached Tuna some twenty miles and another pass short of Guyantse. Tuna was their base for the next three months. Conditions at Tuna, altitude 15,000ft, were grim with intense cold, periodic blizzards and a shortage of fuel. The first casualties of the blizzards were twelve muleteers who developed frost bite. A room in the small local monastery was used as an operating theatre. There is a note that the library had 'pigeon' holes in the walls into which were inserted oblong books made of Chinese paper.

Because of the intense cold and snow thirty men became so incapacitated that they had to be carried out of Tibet on mules. There were over a period seventy-five cases of snow blindness. This condition was intensely painful and so severe that they had to be led out of Tibet. The treeless dusty plain around Tuna produced an epidemic of hacking cough which may have had more to do with the intense cold. On the 23rd February the first case of seven cases of pneumonia is recorded. The rapid fatal clinical course as described raises questions, was this brought on by their dietary privations or because of the temperatures constantly below zero or was it mountain sickness?

Locally grain and meat were available for purchase from the local monasteries, otherwise food had to be carried up or foraged. The leaders of the mission, and the IMS especially were surprised by the poverty of the local Tibetan population which contrasted with the conditions in the monasteries. The mission did what they could to help the local peasants.

On the 17th March they celebrated St Patrick's day, sadly the whiskey was Scotch and not Irish! As the worst of the winter storms passed the happy prospect of moving camp arose. They began to prepare for the next move over the Kangma Pass, 16,000ft, to Guyantse. At this point the first contact with the Tibetan army arose. Their presence had been made known to the mission by the local Tibetans who responded to the generosity shown to them by the mission in general.

A lot of time had been spent in preparatory road work as there were no roads or wheeled vehicles in Tibet. The mission had instructions not to initiate any action, if fired upon they could take necessary action. Their work was interrupted by the appearance of the Tibetan army who were in the process of building a wall across the entrance to the Kangma pass, as the mission force approached they were fired upon and responded, this developed into the action at Guru on the 1st April and a further one at the pass. Between these two actions there were twenty five casualties amongst the mission force. The Tibetans fared far worse with close on seven hundred killed at Guru. Of the 168 Tibetan casualties treated following that action twenty died and the remainder returned to their homes. The Karo La pass 16,000ft at Kangma was blocked by a nine foot stone wall, a recurring feature of the Tibetan's defence. There were Sangrins placed above the wall on the mountain sides, the Tibetans had not allowed for the Gurkas who scaled the mountain and cleared those posts from above. This involved the Gurkas climbing to a height of 18,000Ft.

On the 11th April they reached Guyantse, where over the next three months they experienced constant contact with the Tibetan army. En route to Guyantse they captured 300 sheep. Their route from Tuna had been due north, from Guyantse it was to be north east to Lhasa. To the west of Guyantse was the Monastery of Shigatse whose abbot took an important part in the negotiations. A small village Chung Lo beside the Guyantse river was adapted to provide a secure fortified base for the mission. There was a junction of five rivers at Guyantse and a relief from the arid conditions at Tuna. The subsequent Tibetan strategy was to approach the camp in the early hours attacking before dawn, this caused more inconvenience than injury or loss of life amongst the mission. The principal actions at Guyantse took place between the 12th and 26th May 1904 particularly the capture of the Jong on the 19th and Palla village on the 26th. Of the 43 casulaties there were eight killed and thirty five wounded.

An important action took place at Niani, a village on the mission's supply route from Chumbi, this was in June, by then General Macdonald had brought up a relief party a thousand strong. There were three fortified Tibetan positions: the village, the Jong and the monastery. It was during this that Capt. Kelly was singled out for his bravery and was subsequently awarded a medal. On the 28th June it was found that another monastery Teschen, was unoccupied and presented no threat to the mission. By mid July all Tibetan forces had been cleared out of Guyantse. The march to Lhasa commenced and on the 28th July the Brahmaputra river was crossed and Lhasa reached by the 3rd August where negotiations began. The treaty was signed with the great pomp at the Potola Palace in the presence of the representatives, the Tongsa Penlop for Bhutan, the Chinese envoy and surprisingly the leaders of the annual caravan from Siberia, Mongolia and northern China.

Before this happened Captains Kelly and Cook Young were attacked by a monk wearing chain mail armour who cut them with his sword, wounding both of them though they resisted stoutly. A sentry attacked the lama with his bayonet without any impression, then a Sepoy of the Pioneer corps felled him with a pick axe handle. The lama was tried the next morning and executed.

Was this attack random or did it arise from a misguided belief that the IMS surgeons had offended, by their treatment, the sacred principles of Tibetan medicine which was carried out by the lamas? His monastery were fined 5,000 rupees. As they said they could not pay in cash, barter resulted in rolls of silk for gentlemen and silk Chinese garments for the ladies. These were later sold to great financial benefit!

Sadly the UK Government were not satisfied with Younghusband's treaty which obtained an annual payment of 25,000 rupees a year for twenty five years, although it won the support of the Chinese , it resulted in Bhutan becoming a protectorate and it altered opinions in Nepal.

REFERENCES

1) Seaver G 1952 Francis Younghusband Explorer and Mystic John Murray
2) Chandler E 1905 The unveiling of Lhasa Thos. Nelson & Sons London
3) Ottley W J 1906 With the Mounted Infantry in Tibet Smith Elder and Co
4) Mehra P 1968 The Younghusband Expedition : an Interpretation Asia Publishing House
5) Roll of the Indian Medical Service 1615-1930 Compiled by Lieut Colonel D G 6) 6) Crawford - 1V General list 1897 W Thacker & Co London.
6) Bristol Eye Hospital Committee Records Vol 6 1895/6

Medical Fraud- Causes and Consequences

Some personal reflections

GORDON M. STIRRAT

Emeritus Professor of Obstetrics & Gynaecology and Research Fellow in Ethics in Medicine.

University of Bristol

PRESENTED SEPTEMBER 2012

The serious problem of scientific misconduct in medical research and practice has received considerable publicity in the medical, national and international press particularly in recent years [1-9]. Scientific misconduct is defined as "behaviour by a researcher, intentional or not, that falls short of good ethical and scientific standards" [10]. The National Committees on Scientific Dishonesty in the Nordic Countries have defined the more serious scientific fraud as "intentional distortion of the research process by fabrication of data, text, hypothesis, or methods from another researcher's manuscript form or publication; or distortion of the research process in other ways."[11]

Among the ways that research fraud can arise are:
- Fabrication in which results are made up, then recorded or reported.
- Falsification in which research materials, equipment, or processes are manipulated and/or data or results are changed or omitted such that the research is not accurately represented in the research record.
- Plagiarism in which another person's ideas, processes, results, or words are appropriated without giving due credit
- Suppression in which dissemination and publication of

findings contrary to the interests of some parties (e.g. drug companies) are inhibited.

Research fraud may be perpetrated by an individual (with or without collaborators) or an institution [3]. This paper focuses on the former.

In a Sunday Times article of 12th August 2012 [8], Brian Deer named eight medical or biological scientists and two others who, he alleged, were guilty of serious scientific fraud between 2002 and 2012. A 2009 systematic review [12] reported that around 2% of scientists confessed to committing fraud and 14% were aware of colleagues who had done so. Tavare [4] quotes Malcolm Green, former vice-principal of the Faculty of Medicine, Imperial College, London as saying that "it is highly likely that for every case of fraud that is detected there are a dozen or more that go undetected".

WHAT DRIVES PEOPLE TO INDULGE IN SUCH FRAUD?

From personal experience and reading of the literature I wish to suggest that among the reasons, singly or in combination, are the following:
- A desperate need to succeed because of personal ambition or pressure from more senior staff or sponsors.
- An inability to accept that one may be in error because of 'confirmation bias.' *
- Fear of failure or hubris.
- An overweening need for fame and fortune.
- Personality disorders or psychiatric illness (though this is more frequently claimed post hoc than propter hoc).
- Ineptitude or folly

* (*Confirmation bias* is "the tendency to look at evidence and then try to interpret it to suit our original views" [13].)

In this paper I wish to provide a personal reflection on some of the above causes focussing on two major cases that have impinged on me particularly during my career as a clinical academic.

PERSONAL REFLECTION

In the late 1960s, during my training as an obstetrician, I became aware of a problem that no one seemed to be able to resolve. This is that, having a genetic input from both mother and father, the fetus is at least partly 'foreign' i.e. it is an allograft. Why, therefore, is it not detected by the maternal immune system and rejected? Furthermore, could some pregnancy pathologies (e.g. miscarriage or pre-eclampsia?) have an immunological basis? In November 1979 Hellström et al, cancer immunologists working in Seattle, published a paper in Nature [14] suggesting that not only did the maternal immune system recognise the antigenically foreign embryo but that this immune response was blocked by a serum factor presumed to be 'blocking antibodies'. This was a very significant finding not only for feto-maternal relations but it could also have had important implications for tumour immunology.

I began to pursue this line of research and was able to obtain an MRC grant to do so (those were the days!). In 1971 I was also fortunate enough to obtain a scholarship from the Royal College of Obstetricians and Gynaecologists to visit the Hellströms in the University of Washington in Seattle. On my arrival in Seattle it was disconcerting to discover that they had replaced the technique reported in the Nature article [14] by another.

On my return to St Mary's Hospital in London I began to carry out research in the laboratory while still working as a lecturer in Obstetrics and Gynaecology. I could not get their technique to work so developed my own variant of it [15] on which I worked for the next two years. I still could not reproduce their results. Was this a problem with the method or me; or was this the real situation? Negative findings are always more difficult to sell to the scientific community and examiners of theses! Whatever the cause this was a stressful time and I began to think what I might need to do to come up with some more positive results.

Exactly at that moment in 1974 what became a cause celebre hit the headlines.

THE SLOAN-KETTERING AFFAIR [16]

This was named after the famous cancer research institute in New York in which it occurred. The primary player was William Summerlin, a young dermatologist from Minneapolis. He was carrying out research on skin transplantation in mice and reported that he could transplant tissue from genetically unrelated animals without rejection by the recipient animal if he kept the tissue from the donor in organ culture for four to six weeks. Given that he was working during the time of the Vietnam War, this had tremendous implications for skin grafting of burn victims from that war as well as from other causes. This work came to the attention of Robert A. Good, the famous cancer immunologist, in the Sloan-Kettering Institute. Summerlin went to work with Good in the early 1970's.

Initially Summerlin could not reproduce the results and he claims that Good put him under pressure. The results seemed to improve and on 26 March 1974 he was due to report to Good on the results of the latest experiments. This was a fateful day! A technician noticed that the transplanted patches were actually painted or touched up on the skin of the mice with a felt-tipped marker. When confronted, Summerlin admitted the fraud and other issues emerged later relating to corneal grafts in rabbits.

Summerlin pleaded stress and mental illness and he left to work in obscurity in Louisiana. Robert Good was accused of manipulating national attention and attracting an enormous amount of money for the Institute. Soon afterward he stepped down as director of Sloan-Kettering. This whole episode was described in the New York Times [17] as "a medical Watergate" that reflected "dangerous trends in current efforts to gain scientific acclaim and funds for research. "

There is an interesting codicil to this story. One of the mice in the original experiments in which the skin graft had survived was still alive. When tested it was found not to be pure bred but a hybrid. At the time I recall being told anecdotally that a lab technician in the original laboratory had allowed some of the pure bred mice to escape and had hastily tried to put them back in their cages without confessing this at the time. This cannot now be confirmed but if mice of different strains had been mixed they would interbreed and produce hybrid offspring. The original success may have been due to the actions of the lab technician rather than any intent to commit fraud by Dr Summerlin. Unfortunately he became trapped by this pseudo success. For me this was a wake up call and, in 1975, I reported my findings, 'warts and all', in my MD thesis.

On moving to Oxford University in 1975, I was subsequently part of a research team that was among the first to demonstrate that the fetus was protected against rejection by very special properties of the placenta and not by 'blocking antibodies' at all [18].

Interestingly it is the placenta that provides the link to the second story I wish to tell.

THE FRAUD OF ABDERHALDEN'S ENZYMES [19]

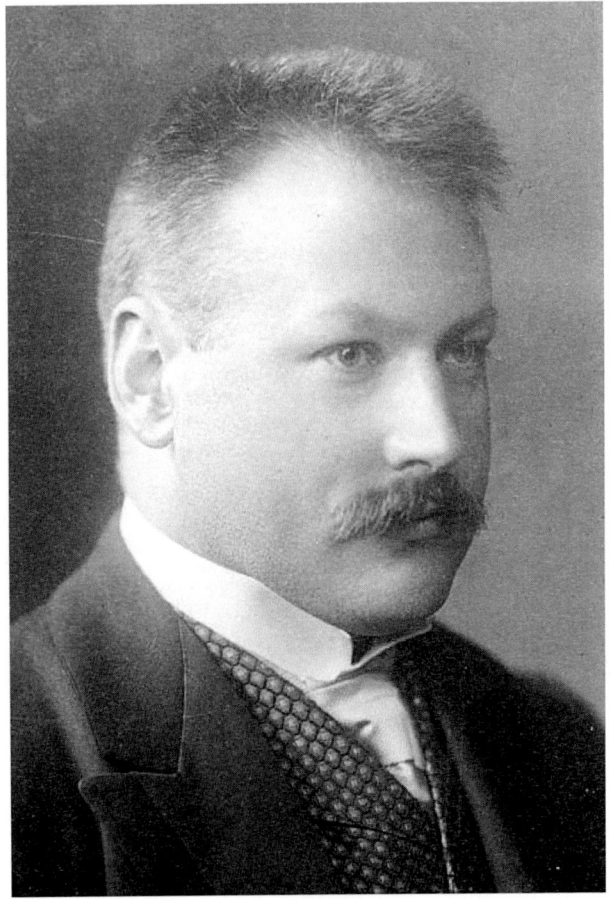

Figure 1
Emil Abderhalden (1877-1950) as a young man
(Wikipedia)

Emil Abderhalden, born in Switzerland in 1877, has been called the founder of scientific biochemistry. He was Professor of Physiology and Physiological Chemistry in Halle University, Germany, from 1911 to his death in 1950. Interestingly, in light of subsequent events, he edited the journal 'Ethik' from 1922 to 1935 and was president of the Leopoldina, Germany's oldest Academy of Science, between 1931and 1946. He was author of more than 1000 research papers though his scientific approach was interesting - he once told an eminent immunologist "if an experiment worked well once why should it be repeated?" [19] Actively anti-semitic, he was also a convinced eugenicist [19].

In 1909 he reported a discovery that he considered to be the most important of his long career. This was of 'abwehrfermente' (defence or protection enzymes) that were produced by a process that started with boiling a placenta. Among the suggested uses of their detection were the diagnosis of pregnancy, cancers, infectious diseases such as syphilis and psychiatric diseases such as schizophrenia.

By 1914 there were 451 papers enthusiastically describing various uses of the test for abwehrfermente and Abderhalden suggested that "cancer treatment using abwehrfermente is just around the corner" without giving any information as to the mechanism for this. However, also in 1914 Michaelis and Lagermark [20] published a paper stating that they could not repeat Abderhalden's experiments. This was the end of Michaelis's career in Germany. Belief in the value of testing for abwehrfermente persisted. In 1942 the test was used to demonstrate supposed racial differences in responses to infectious diseases and in 1943 Verschuer and Mengele obtained a grant from Deutsche Forschungsgemeinschaft to test the production of these enzymes in response to deliberate infections of over 200 individuals of various races [19]. These tests took place in Auschwitz.

Emil Abderhalden died in 1950 but his son Rudolf continued with his father's work. He declared that abwehrfermente were *"the perfect diagnostic tools to determine the optimal cell type for 'fresh cell therapy'"* [19] (another medical fraud!)

Despite their non-existence papers on the subject did not

disappear from the literature until the 1960s and fresh cell therapy was outlawed in Germany only in 1997. Deichmann & Muller-Hill [19] ask *"How could Abderhalden continue with the deception from 1915 until his death in 1950? His strategy was simple and straightforward. He must have had collaborators who found what he wanted them to find. In medical biochemistry, ideas or hope may be stronger than experimentally proven reality".*

Recent literature already referred to [1-9] suggests that this chilling tale has counterparts in modern science and medicine.

WHAT ARE THE CONSEQUENCES OF MEDICAL FRAUD?

In the above stories some of the consequences of medical fraud have been explicit and others implicit. Among them are that it:
- Directly or indirectly harms patients [2,5]. False hopes or unwarranted alarm may be generated.
- Distorts the evidence base
- Misdirects research efforts
- Wastes funds
- Destroys careers both of the perpetrators, their associates and, sometimes, 'whistle blowers'.
- Damages public trust in Science

It is, therefore, important that effective action be taken to prevent scientific misconduct and fraud. In 1989 the National Institute of Health in the USA established the Office of Scientific Integrity though it has been described as 'Orwellian' [21]. The independent UK Research Integrity Office, established in 2006, aims to promote the good governance, management and conduct of academic, scientific and medical research; share good practice on how to address poor practice, misconduct and unethical behaviour; and give confidential, independent and expert advice on specific research projects, cases, problems and issues [22]. In 2009 it published a Code of Practice for Research [23]. In addition, on 11 July 2012, Universities UK launched a concordat to strengthen research integrity of government departments. It remains to be seen how effective these measures really are but further consideration is beyond the scope of this paper.

REFERENCES

1. Evered D, Lazar P. Misconduct in medical research. Lancet 1995; 345: 1161-2
2. Godlee F. The fraud behind the MMR scare. BMJ 2011; 342:d22
3. Godlee F. Institutional research misconduct BMJ 2011; 343: d7284
4. Tavare A Managing research misconduct. Is anyone getting it right? BMJ 2011; 343:d8212
5. Godlee F. Research misconduct harms patients. BMJ 2012; 344: e-14
6. Godlee F, Wager E. Research misconduct in the UK BMJ 2012; 344: d8357.
7. Tavare A, Godless F. Tackling research misconduct BMJ 2012; 345 :e5402
8. Deer B Doctoring the evidence: What the science establishment doesn't want you to know. Sunday Times 12 August 2012.
9. Riis P Scientific dishonesty: European reflections. J Clin Pathol 2001; 541: 4-6
10. Nimmo WS, ed. Misconduct in biomedical research: final consensus statement. In: Joint consensus conference on misconduct in biomedical research. Proc R Coll Physicians Edinb; 2000; 30(suppl 7):2.
11. Nylenna, M et al. Handling of scientific dishonesty in the Nordic countries. National Committees on Scientific Dishonesty in the Nordic Countries. Lancet 1999; 354: 57–61
12. Fanelli D. How many scientists fabricate and falsify research? A systematic review and meta-analysis of survey data. PloS One 2009;4: e5738
13. Aaronovitch D. The Stalinists of the mind are alive and well. Sunday Times 23 August 2012 p.21.
14. Hellstrom KE. Hellstrom I, Brawn J Abrogation of cellular immunity to antigenically foreign mouse embryonic cells by a serum factor. Nature 1969; 224:914-5
15. Stirrat GM. A terminal-labelling microcytotoxicity assay with 125I-iododeoxyuridine as a label for target cells. J.Immunol. Methods 1976; 12:201-8.
16. Culliton BJ. The Sloan-Kettering Affair Science 1974; 184; 1154-7.
17. Brody JE. Charge of False Research Data Stirs Cancer Scientists at Sloan-Kettering New York Times April 18 1974
18. Sunderland CA, Naim M et al The expression of MHC antigens by human chorionic villi. J. Reprod Immunol 1981; 3: 323.
19. Deichmann U, Muller-Hill B. The Fraud of Abderhalden's Enzymes Nature 1998; 393: 109-111

20. Michaelis, L. & Lagermark, Lv. Bedeutung der Abderhalden'schen Untersuchungsmethode. Deutsche Med. Wochenschr. 1914; 7: 316–319
21. Klein DF. Should the government assure scientific integrity? Academic Medicine 1993: 68 (9 suppl.) S56-9
22. UK Research Integrity Office http://www.ukrio.org/ accessed 13 September 2012.
23. Code of Practice for Research: Promoting good practice and preventing misconduct. UKRIO 2009 http://www.ukrio.org/what-we-do/code-of-practice-for-research/ accessed 13 September 2012.

The Junior Doctors' Dispute 1975

Paul Goddard
Visiting Professor UWE
Former Treasurer and Vice-President JHDA
Presented June 2013

THE HISTORICAL SETTING

Britain's sterling was the world's reserve currency until after the Second World War. In 1967 the unthinkable happened... the Labour government devalued sterling by 14%. Ted Heath's Conservative government was in power from 1970 to 1974 but industrial action by the coal miners brought the country to a standstill and a three-day week was instigated to conserve electricity and, for the same reason, television companies were required to cease broadcasting at 10.30pm [1]. Hospitals continued to work normally throughout the three-day week thus providing no relief for the overworked junior doctors, many of whom were expected to put in more than one hundred hours a week.

In 1974 there were two general elections in the United Kingdom. In February no party won an overall majority but in October the Labour party, led by Harold Wilson, won by three seats. In London the IRA were busy bombing innocent victims.

THE NATIONAL HEALTH SERVICE

Throughout 1974 and 1975 storm clouds were gathering for the NHS. The angry red queen, Barbara Castle, was firmly in charge of the Department of Health and Social Security (DHSS). As it says in the authorized biography of her life Barbara Castle's '..final act on the Westminster stage was her boldest, her most political and her least successful.' [2]

She set out to improve on Bevan's NHS by taking on the doctors in two major disputes. The one that she set most store by was the Paybed Dispute but simultaneously she found herself and the country embroiled in a dispute with the junior doctors.

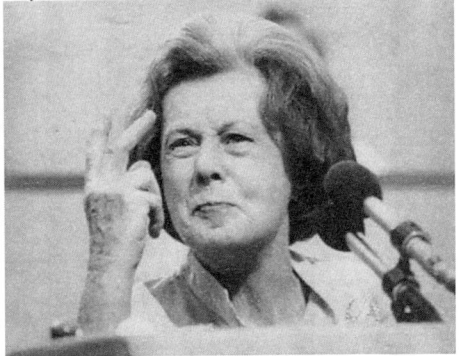

Figure 1
The angry red Queen: Barbara Castle
(The image was provided by the copyright holder for use in the Cotton Town digitisation project)

CASTLE'S OPPONENTS

Her major opponents were Mr. (later Sir) Anthony Grabham chairman of the consultants' committee of the British Medical Association (BMA) and Elinor Kapp of the Junior Hospital Doctors' Association (JHDA). About Grabham, Barbara Castle wrote in her diary that there was *'no doubting Grabham's mood of barely restrained viciousness'* and *'with Grabham they had a fanatic in charge'*. [3] Writing about the softly spoken and very reasonable Dr. Kapp of the JHDA, Castle called her *'their militant chairman.'* [3].

CASTLE'S ALLIES

Castle's allies included:
- The Unions
- The Labour party, especially David Owen and Jack Straw
- The battling Granny
- Some members of the Junior Committee of the BMA

The Unions were very left wing. The most powerful union leader in the 1970s was Jack Jones, General Secretary of the TGWU. After Jones died in 2009, Christopher Andrew's official history of MI5 confirmed that Jones was knowingly a KGB agent. [4]
David Owen (now the Right Honourable the Lord Owen) was Minister of State for Health from July 1974.
Jack Straw, a Labour councillor for Islington in 1975, had previously been an extremely left wing NUS president (69-71) and before that had been branded a *"troublemaker acting with malice aforethought"* by the Foreign Office having disrupted a student trip to Chile. [5]
The battling Granny was the name given by the press to Medical Secretary Mrs Esther Brookstone, local steward of the National Union of Public Employees (NUPE) at the new Charing Cross hospital. As an old communist who had worked for Harry Pollit, the Communist Party of Great Britain (CPGB) General Secretary, she brought the hospital to a standstill against private beds on the 15th floor. Harry Pollit always supported Stalin. Pre-war Castle had entertained Pollit. Also we must consider Michael Foot, Secretary of State for Employment in 1975 and later leader of the Labour Party. Foot received money regularly from the KGB 'for the Tribune' and was considered by the KGB to be an agent or confidential contact.[6]
In 1974 the junior doctors had pressed for a forty hour contract with overtime in line with normal practice for other employees.

This led to the Junior Doctors' Dispute.

The junior doctors wanted a new contract because working night and day as a junior doctor was becoming almost unbearable for many of them. This had not previously been the case. My father-in-law remembered his time as a houseman with a nostalgic fondness. He had worked unpaid and lived-in but there were no cardiac arrest bleeps, few drips, little work at night and a good mess atmosphere. In comparison I worked 120 hours a week, covered casualty at night, never had an undisturbed night in the first six months I was working and considered myself lucky to get an hour of continuous sleep. And to cap it all the administration were trying to close the Doctors' Mess.

Junior doctors were entitled to claim at "time plus a quarter" after eighty hours. But many consultants would not sign the Extra Duty Award (EDA) forms. So Juniors wanted a contract that did not require payment to be claimed in that way. Barbara Castle agreed to a forty hours contract so in early 1975 the BMA signed for the contract unpriced. On January 8th 1975 Barbara Castle met the Junior Doctors from the BMA. She wrote in her diary..."*The junior hospital doctors turn out to be nice, young, reasonable chaps*" and "*they would go to the Review Body arguing for a hefty overtime rate, while we would go and argue for a modest one.*"[3] But secretly she had decided to take unfair advantage of the junior doctors' good nature. She was heard in the corridors of power saying "*I will take the Junior Hospital Doctors to the cleaners.*" (Conversation relayed to the author in early 1975 by a civil servant [7]).

Meanwhile Barbara Castle was very ambitious and was particularly keen to stay on the National Executive of the Labour party and to be the darling of the Labour movement. To do this Castle needed to keep the unions and the TUC on her side. COHSE and NUPE, the public service unions, wanted to get rid of the paybeds. Thus for doctrinaire reasons Castle had become determined to rid the NHS of paybeds, come what may [2,3]. She believed that her disputes with the doctors would prove to the party faithful how true she was to left wing ideals.

Castle's official were appalled at the idea because of the cost implications. They would lose somewhere between 25 and 50 million pounds on a budget of £3.3 billion ... at a time when inflation had hit 26.9%!

COHSE and NUPE agreed to stick to the Government's pay policy if the Pay Beds bill was introduced. BUT ... the TUC would not agree that more money could be spent on the junior hospital doctors' contract.

That sets the scene. Having heard the Castle quote about junior doctors from a civil servant I realised that the new contract would prove to be a problem.

THE PRICING

Indeed, when the junior's contract was priced it was dire:

- 40 hours for basic salary
- 4 hours free (thus automatically turning it into a 44 hour contract)
- From 44 hours most juniors would be on 10% of the basic salary hourly rate. Not time plus 10%....just 10%.
- A few would be on 30% of the basic salary hourly rate
- One third of doctors would lose money and the effect would be the opposite to that intended by the medical negotiators... it would be cheaper to employ fewer doctors for longer hours since working the juniors even harder carried no financial penalty and considerable financial advantage.

I immediately joined the BMA and the JHDA, became a BMA local representative and treasurer of the JHDA.

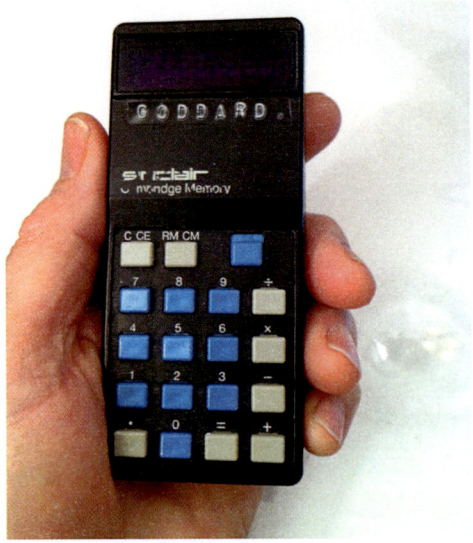

Figure 2 The author's Sinclair Calculator

I then sat with my Sinclair calculator and worked through all the figures becoming convinced that the intention was to actually save money from the doctors' pay budget.

This I announced to the press but it was roundly refuted by the BMA as well as by the Labour Government. The DHSS surprisingly offered an audit of doctors' pay but this was rejected by the BMA.

I was taken down to the Houses of Parliament to lobby my MP. Instead I saw David Owen and impressed on him that the Junior Doctors were being treated unfairly and it would lead to a long period of industrial action.

According to the Castle Diaries the BMA met Barbara Castle on 20th Oct 1975.[3]

The representatives of the Junior Doctors were Mander, Ford and Bell.

Mander told Castle that the detriment situation was unacceptable. Junior Doctors around the country would not tolerate having their pay cut. Ford, according to the diaries, was *'clearly desperately anxious for a settlement'* [3], Grabham was *'obviously annoyed at the rapport which was building between (Barbara Castle) and the juniors.'* [3]

Castle wrote about the meeting *'Not too bad at all. Ford and Bell are clearly doing their best for us , though we learned (later) that Mander ...resigned'* [3]

Elinor Kapp of the JHDA accepted the offer of an audit but the DHSS then refused to do it and put a D notice on doctors' pay stating that it was against national security for the press to write about it!

At this point doctors voted through the JHDA for industrial action. This would consist of forty hours work to rule or even complete walk out depending on the hospital involved. Barbara Castle and the BMA both flatly refused to meet Elinor Kapp and the JHDA.

'Elinor Kapp and her militant men of the JHDA have continued to let off fireworks at the fringe of all this, furious because the BMA won't agree to include them in negotiations' [3].

At this point I was invited to talk to the Current Affairs meeting of the London School of Economics.

THE LONDON SCHOOL OF ECONOMICS

Doctors were perceived by the left wing as being resolutely conservative. The LSE was not going to be an easy place to put our case.

I prepared a poster. On one side it stated:

Not a penny less, Not an hour more
1926, Miners' strike and General Strike

On the other side the message was very similar:

Not a penny less. Not an hour more Junior Doctors' Dispute 1975

The attendees at the LSE Current Affairs meeting found it hard to understand that I was referring to 10% or 30% of time rate not time rate plus 10%. After overcoming that difficulty three post grad students were assigned to help me. The role of the JHDA and the ongoing dispute became the subject matter of their theses.
- Bernard Casey
- Alan Cave
- Peter Martin

Many meetings were held at the LSE resulting in political and media pressure on the government.

Now the Consultants started a work to rule over the Paybeds dispute joining the Juniors who were still working to rule over their contract dispute.

The JHDA were finally allowed to meet officials of the DHSS and the Department agreed to hold the audit.

The audit agreed that the figure had been wrong leading to some mirth in political circles. Barbara Castle was now under considerable strain and was becoming the butt of jokes in the media.

Castle to Wilson: **'Oh silly me! I got my sums wrong about the doctors' pay! I shall tell them that I can't count'**
Wilson (aside): **'I've already told them she doesn't count'**
Sun Cartoon December 1975

The Junior Doctors' Dispute 1975

But the extra money was not sufficient to get rid of the detriment problem. At this point the LSE suggested that the number of hours worked by doctors might be presented as fewer than originally calculated thus allowing more pay per hour. The sum of money would thus be divided by a smaller figure as in the simple equation below.

$$\text{Pay per hour} = \frac{\text{Sum of money}}{\text{Number of hours}}$$

When the contract was re-priced the 4 hour free period was removed, the 10% level was removed and 30% was agreed for all overtime.

The result was that the doctors' overtime did not cost the £10m secretly planned, nor the £12m the DHSS had stated publicly, or even the £14.2m from the audit or £18m, I believed had previously been spent. The sum spent was £30.5million in the first year alone. This increase from the planned £10m to £30.5m would be equivalent to at least £200 to £300 million in today's money.

CONCLUSION

The doctors' disputes broke the career of Barbara Castle and Margaret Thatcher became the first female prime minister, not the angry red queen. Industrial action served to show the serious intent of the doctors and the fact that we still looked after emergencies kept the public on our side. The media were important in creating pressure on the Government and the LSE were very helpful behind the scenes.

It is doubtful that industrial action alone would have persuaded the DHSS to pay doctors more since the NHS did not run like any normal business. Cancelling work just saved money in the NHS of 1975. Careful analysis of the figures was very important. The junior doctors are again in dispute with the Government, this time a Conservative one. Once again the Government want poorly paid doctors to work longer and more antisocial hours for no more pay and in some cases for less. It is a mistake on the part of the Conservatives to enter into such a fight with a group of people who are so admired by the public.

The junior doctors would be sensible to find out whether or not working to rule or striking costs the hospitals money. The system is now run differently and the withdrawal of some elective work may create greater pressure on the management than other work. Alternatively if it is not costing the NHS money when the doctors' withdraw their labour it might actually be better to insist on doing the work and doing so to the best of their ability in line with all of the GMC guidelines. This "working perfectly" could be much more expensive to the NHS and thus put more pressure on Government. The junior doctors may require assistance in working out the best way of doing this and also how to present themselves to the public. Perhaps the LSE will help again?

In the meantime the Government should consider that the real problem with the NHS right now is not the lack of 24 hour cover, the doctors already provide that. The pressing conundrum is how to renegotiate the Private Finance Initiative (PFI) contracts that are bleeding the hospitals dry. These are the fault of Blair and Brown but Cameron has to deal with them. They were never in the best interests of the NHS or the people of the UK and unless the contracts are altered many of the hospitals will soon move completely into the ownership of the PFI private business partners. That would, indeed, spell the end of the NHS.

REFERENCES

1. https://en.wikipedia.org/wiki/Three-Day_Week
2. Red Queen, the authorized biography of Barbara Castle, by Anne Perkins. Pan Books 2004.
3. The Castle Diaries 1964-1976 Macmillan 1990
4. The Defence of the Realm: The Authorized History of MI5. Allen Lane. 2009. ISBN 0-7139-9885-7. (hardcover)
5. http://news.bbc.co.uk/1/hi/uk_politics/5228770.stm
6. http://www.telegraph.co.uk/comment/columnists/charlesmoore/7377111/Was-Foot-a-national-treasure-or-the-KGBs-useful-idiot.html
7. Personal communication early 1975

Francis Galton

A passion for measurement

DR MARTIN CROSFILL

Presented September 2013

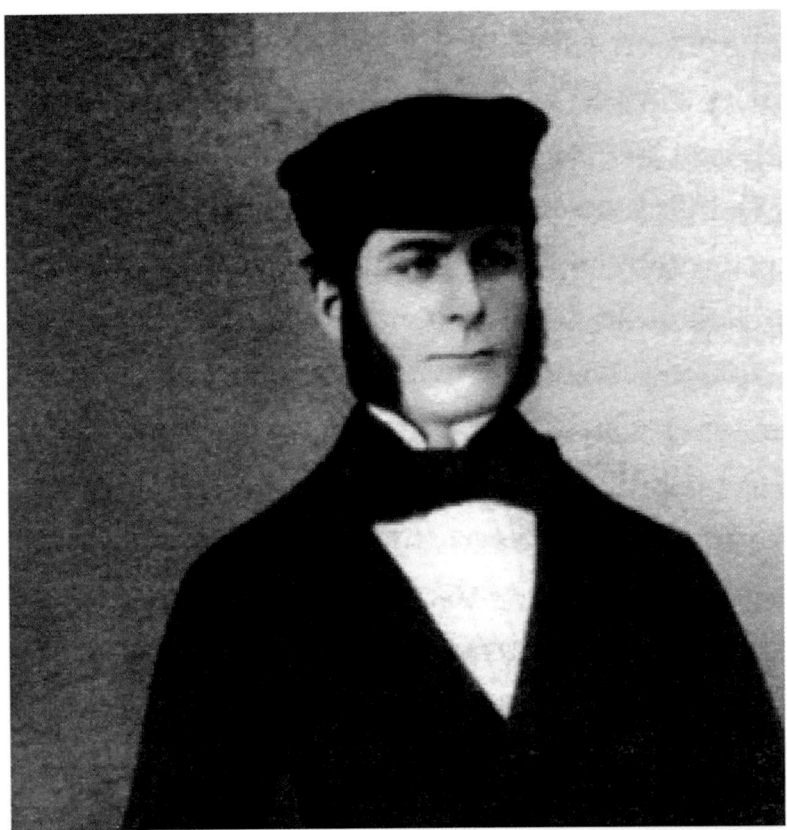

Figure 1. Francis Galton as a young man

My first introduction to Francis Galton was in a scholarly work called "Eccentric Doctors". Apparently he believed that, in order to function properly, the brain should be prevented from overheating, to which end he devised a 'ventilating hat' controlled by a rubber bulb. When in company he would ask permission to wear this lest he embarrass the guests by falling in a fit on the floor.

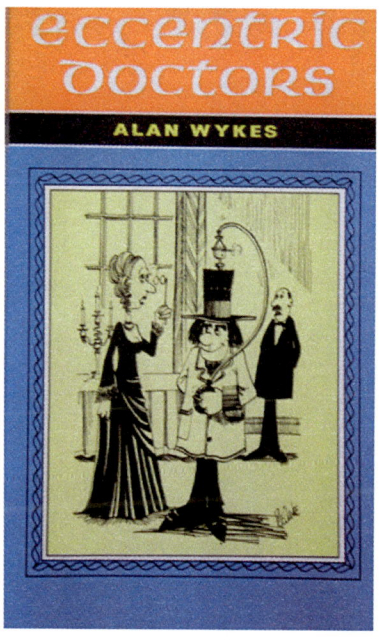

Figure 2.
Eccentric Doctors

Clearly one needed to know more and, indeed, more there was. For anyone whose overriding interest became the relationship between Nature and Nurture, his family provided plenty of material.

Both his grandfathers were members of the Lunar Society. Samuel Galton, his paternal grandfather was an FRS who demonstrated the role of the primary colours in the production of white light; he was also that ultimate oxymoron, a Quaker arms manufacturer. From his mother's side came physical stamina in the shape of a great uncle who was renowned for walking 1000 miles in 100 days – in a onesey! More importantly, his paternal grandfather was Erasmus Darwin, physician, inventor, poet, the classic eighteenth century polymath.

The Lunar Society included such names as Joseph Priestley, Matthew Boulton, James Watt and Josiah Wedgewood. The society was as much social as scientific and it is not surprising that we find marital alliances, Darwins with Galtons, Boultons with Watts, Wedgewoods with Darwins. Two generations down, connections are still close. Charles Darwin was Francis Galton's cousin, albeit twice removed, whilst Matthew Watt Boulton was a schoolmate and Montagu, his brother a travelling companion. Such were the ramifications of the Society that Galton's parents, Samuel 'Tertius' and Violetta Darwin lived in a house built by another member, William Withering of digitalis fame. The house was on land previously owned by Joseph Priestley whose own dwelling and laboratory had been trashed and burned by the mob in 1791. Here in 1822 Francis was born, the youngest of seven surviving children. The four oldest were girls and they vied with each other to have the honour of looking after the new baby. Their mother was probably only too happy to cede the responsibility, which was conferred on Adele ("Delly") the second eldest. Adele had suffered from birth from a spinal deformity which, for much of her time, confined her to the couch; this facilitated five years of intensive nurture with the result that he was able to say that:

"*by the age of four I can read any English book, I can say all the Latin substantives and adjectives and active verbs beside fifty two lines of Latin poetry.. I can cast up any sums in addition and can multiply by 2345678 and 10. I can also say the pence table and I know the clock.*"

By five he knew the works of Homer which he re-enacted whilst riding his horse in the fields around the house. In spite of his pressure cooking he was an active little boy with an interest in wildlife and in gardening.

School proved an eye opener; he was startled to find that his fellow pupils had never even heard of Homer, let alone read him. He had a habit of producing literary quotations at appropriate moments and in later life admitted that he must have seemed a bit of a prig. Two further schools followed and then he was sent to King Edward's Grammar School in Birmingham, which proved to be a melange of Latin, Greek and the birch. His diary at this time reads;

Saturday. Bought a cat's gallows. Got caned
Monday Got caned.

On another occasion a schoolmaster chastised eleven members of his class for mispronunciation; in an early manifestation of his lifelong passion for measurement, Galton timed him. It took eight minutes.

He left school at sixteen and it was decided that he should study medicine. His introduction to the subject was by way of an attachment to a chemist's in Birmingham and then by shadowing the local GP in Leamington. It was here he saw his first autopsy – that of a young serving girl who had succumbed to a gastric perforation. Galton's comment showed his wide reading and extraordinary memory for apposite quotations, this from Richard the Second:

"Death....................with a little pin bores through the castle wall and...........Farewell King!"

This was not the end of his introductory course, for he embarked on a European tour in the company of two senior medical students. The ostensible purpose was to visit German hospitals but predictably there were many diversions and if he came away with anything, it was with a love for travelling.

In September 1838 medical life started in earnest as a pupil at the Birmingham General. His autobiography gives a vivid and amusing account of hospital life but also illustrates his ability to think 'outside the box'. He notes, for example, that the stethoscope was little used, possibly because the consultants were a little deaf. He wonders whether *'youths of sharp hearing should ......be used.......... as pointers or setters'* –as a sort of human amplifier. Of more contemporary interest was a suggestion that:

'It is to be wished that some "Index of Curative Skill" could be awarded to doctors, based on their respective hospital successes. If it could be compiled truthfully, it would be an excellent guide to those who wanted a doctor but were doubtful whom to consult. A high index of curative skill would serve as a measure of merit, and the fee to the doctor might be regulated by its height.'

Along the same lines was the notion:

'Suppose two different and conflicting treatments of a particular malady; let the patients suffering from it be given the option of being placed under Dr A or Dr B..... .and the results be statistically compared'

Part of his learning process was to test the effects of drugs upon himself, to which end he started at the letter A in the pharmacopoeia and worked his way through. He got no further than C for Croton oil whereupon he probably felt he had learned enough. A year at Kings College Hospital proved to be more quietly academic and offered more in the way of a social life. His cousin, Charles Darwin had just returned from his voyaging and it was the latter who persuaded him to interrupt his medical studies and take a mathematical degree. He had successfully completed his preclinical examinations and so, with the reluctant consent of his parents he took up a place at Trinity College Cambridge, although not before he had made another foreign trip, this time reaching Istanbul.

He flung himself wholeheartedly into student life and there

are various tales of his escapades, including his entry into a cage of lions, from which he miraculously emerged unscathed. He also gained a reputation as an inventor, creating a number of items which became known as Galton's toys. Academically however he struggled; he worked prodigiously long hours and, in order to stay awake, devised a 'gumption-reviver' to combat this, consisting of a cold water drip onto his betowelled head. His gyp's task was to replenish the reservoir every quarter of an hour. It was to no avail; he missed time through illness in his first year and although he struggled through the second year he never gained more than a second class pass and eventually suffered a mental breakdown at the beginning of his third year. He now settled for an ordinary pass ('Poll') degree which freed him to enjoy to the full the wider aspects of university life.

After leaving Cambridge, the original plan was for him to resume his medical studies in London, but his father's death in 1844 relieved him of this obligation; furthermore he was now rich. What follow are described by one biographer as *'the wilderness years'*. During this time he managed to fit in an adventurous and mildly hedonistic trip which took him as far as Khartoum and thence to Damascus. Much of this time was spent enjoying field sports but he did manage to publish the description of a teleprinter, he called it a "Telotype", which was some fifty years ahead of its time.

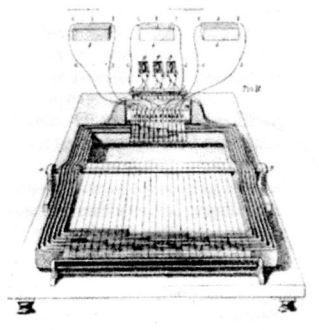

Figure 3. Galton's Telotype

By the late 1840's Galton was beginning to feel restless; whether it was the lure of big game hunting or whether the stories of heroic explorations that were filling the newspapers bolstered his resolve, he now determined to lead an expedition to Africa.. Using his connections to the full, he obtained official endorsement from the Royal Geographical Society for his trip. This eased the bureaucratic burden although the financing and planning were all down to Galton.

The expedition was highly successful; he proved himself to be a resourceful, courageous leader and diplomatist. His mapping and daily scientific observations were meticulous and valuable, if occasionally wayward. His interest in the human form led him to record the dimensions of a particularly steatopygous Hottentot lady, Mrs Petrus. Not wishing to embarrass her by running a tape measure over her, he asked her to pose by a tree and, from a discreet distance, obtained her measurements by triangulation, using his sextant.

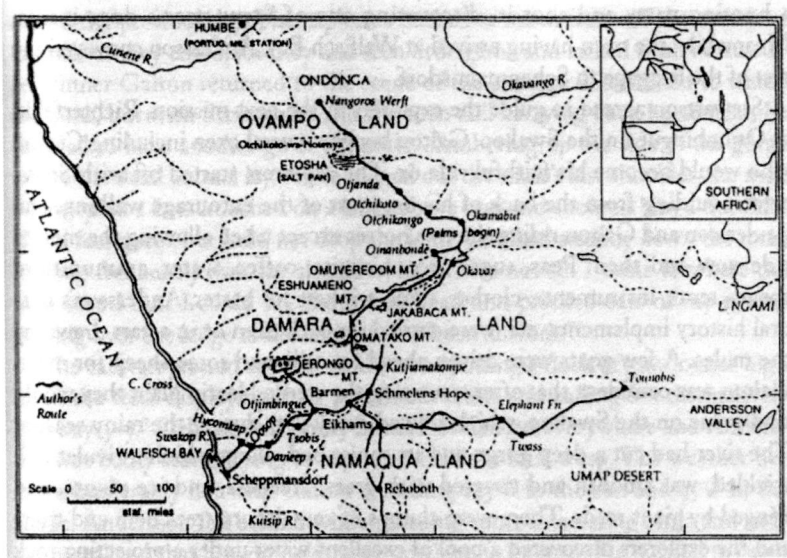

Figure 4.
A map from the highly successful expedition to Africa

On his return to England he found himself a celebrity and a deserving winner of the RGS's Gold Medal. He wrote several accounts of his adventures and one, "The Art of Travel" is still in print.

Galton married in August 1853 and spent the rest of the year honeymooning in Italy, France and Spain. A liking for extended foreign holidays became a feature of their life together. It took Galton a whole year to recover from his African journey and he whiled away his time by experimenting with a specially adapted teapot in order to discover how to make the perfect cuppa. It turns out that the water in the pot must be maintained at 180-190°F for eight minutes. The formula $C=n(e-t)/(t-1)$ is somehow relevant. He next applied his mind to calculating the total volume of gold in the world – his solution was 3053 cu ft. He was surprised to realise that it would all have fitted into his drawing room.

Eccentricities apart, Galton was fast becoming a member of the establishment He was made a Fellow of the Royal Society in 1856, joined the Athenaeum and became secretary of the RGS in 1857. The following year he joined the management committee of Kew Observatory. From this point on, even Galton, in his memoirs, found himself unable to make chronological sense of his biography.

In 1861, following Captain Fitzroy's publicly humiliating attempt to forecast the weather (and his subsequent suicide) he realised that what was lacking was knowledge of contemporaneous continental if not global weather patterns. He therefore wrote to meteorologists all over Europe asking for data on wind direction and speed, barometric pressure and so on, information to be obtained at specified dates and times in December of that year. The data showed that a depression centred over Northern Europe with the winds circling round it in an anticlockwise fashion. This was the opposite of what was known to happen in a cyclone, for which reason Galton coined the term anticyclone. He continued

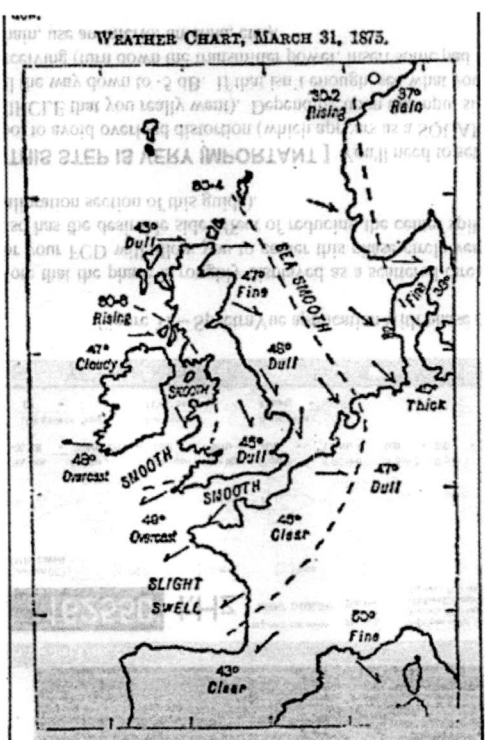

Figure 5. Weather map 1875

to collect data over the next few years until, on April 1st 1875 he provided the Times with its first ever weather map. .

In 1859 , his cousin, Charles Darwin published "The Origin of Species" an event which was to prove a turning point in his life. In his own words *"This marked an epoch in my own mental development."* Typically he took evolutionary theory several stages down the line and began to consider how this knowledge could be used actually to improve the human race. The idea of selective breeding for physical traits was understood, after all it had long been applied to domesticated animals, but the concept that mental characteristics could similarly be influenced was totally new. His first publication on the subject *"Hereditary Talent* and *Character"* was in Macmillan's Magazine, but it was not until 1869, when *"Hereditary Genius"* appeared, that he attempted to put a scientific gloss on his theory. He began by demonstrating that the normal distribution, what we now term the bell curve, applied to human measurement – height for example. He then made the imaginative leap to assume that it also applied to talent. He did this in several ways, for example by plotting out the exam results of Sandhurst cadets. He next attempts to satisfy himself that reputation implies ability. It is an article of faith, of course, that ability is inherited. He expressed his creed thus;

"I have no patience with the hypothesis occasionally expressed, and often implied, that babies are born pretty much alike, and that the sole agencies in creating differences between man and boy, and man and man are steady application and effort. It is in the most unqualified manner that I object to pretensions of natural equality."

To support his thesis he compiled a database obtained, for example, from the Times obituary columns and various reference books, among them a "Dictionary of Men of our Time" to identify those men (always men) of outstanding ability – one in 4000 according to his calculations. These he divides into various categories, judges, generals, scientists, divines and so on. He then investigates their families to prove that there is a higher than expected incidence of similar ability the closer the relationship to the subject.

The book was received by the critics with somewhat sceptical ambivalence, thus showing themselves more scientific than the scientists who approved it. The divines, who had come out rather badly in the survey, were predictably opposed, the more so when Galton published an essay on the lack of efficacy of prayer, pointing out that the Royal Family, who were prayed for weekly in the churches, showed no greater longevity than the rest of us. His wife, who was deeply religious, persuaded him to drop the subject. For the remainder of his life Galton occupied himself with the measurement of different attributes of man. He attempted to counter some of his critics in a short tract *"English Men of Science, their Nature and Nurture"*. His coinage of this now famous phrase may owe its origin to Shakespeare, whose works he knew intimately (Tempest 1V i.). The work was based on the results of a seven page psychological questionnaire, submitted to 192 Fellows of the Royal Society. Astonishingly over ninety returns were available for analysis. The results may have been somewhat inconclusive, but the method used was novel and has served since as a useful investigative tool. Another "first" that came from this investigation, and a further example of Galton's lateral thinking, was the subject of twin studies. Although, for lack of material, he did not pursue this, he nevertheless laid the foundation for much further work. His passionate desire to quantify every conceivable attribute of the human race, physical and psychological, led him at times into blind alleys, some of them distinctly murky; his opinion of the native African would land him in court today.

Skull and facial measurements were much in vogue following the work of Lombroso, Bertillon and he had himself "Bertillonized" as earlier he had been phrenologised. He attempted to define the characteristics of the average criminal by a method of composite photography. Unfortunately the average criminal looked remarkably like the average bank clerk. He did however devise a way of measuring the profile so that the coordinates of the facial characteristics could be transmitted, for example by telegraph, to distant police forces. His continuing work on the bodily characteristics of criminals gave rise, indirectly, to his book "Fingerprints", the first systematic summary of the subject. If he was going to quantify talent he needed to obtain some measure of the quality of the mind. He began by writing a number of words on cards and checking the time it took him to think of an associated idea. Needless to say he invented a machine to measure reaction time. These word association experiments took him into some odd corners of his own psyche, some of which he was reluctant to acknowledge, so he extended his researches by means of one of his questionnaires, this time on the subject of mental imagery. To his disappointment, his scientific friends struggled with this but the general public proved better at visualising and even provided some examples of synaesthesia. His psychological studies were brought together in 1883 in *"Inquiries into Human Faculty"*. This book is noted for the first use of the word Eugenics. Galton believed with increasingly passionate, almost religious enthusiasm, that the human race could be "bettered" by appropriate breeding – that the talented (i.e. successful) should be encouraged to marry early and breed copiously, whereas those whom he did not hesitate to call idiots and degenerates should be discouraged, forcibly if necessary.

In the meantime, these beliefs required the backing of science. His already enormous database was augmented by information from an anthropometric laboratory which he set up first at the International Health Exhibition, later at the South Kensington museum. Its lineal descendant is the Galton Institute at University College. The venture proved popular – participants (who included Gladstone) paid to be tested and measured and, latterly, to record their fingerprints. Other measurements included the strength of a blow and the highest frequency. This was estimated using Galton's whistle, an instrument which remained in the catalogues until the coming of the audiometer. All this was brought together in 1889 in what is possibly his most important publication *"Natural Inheritance."* The book is a useful contribution to the science of heredity and groundbreaking in its use of statistics. Among his many contributions are the notions of regression to the mean and of correlation.

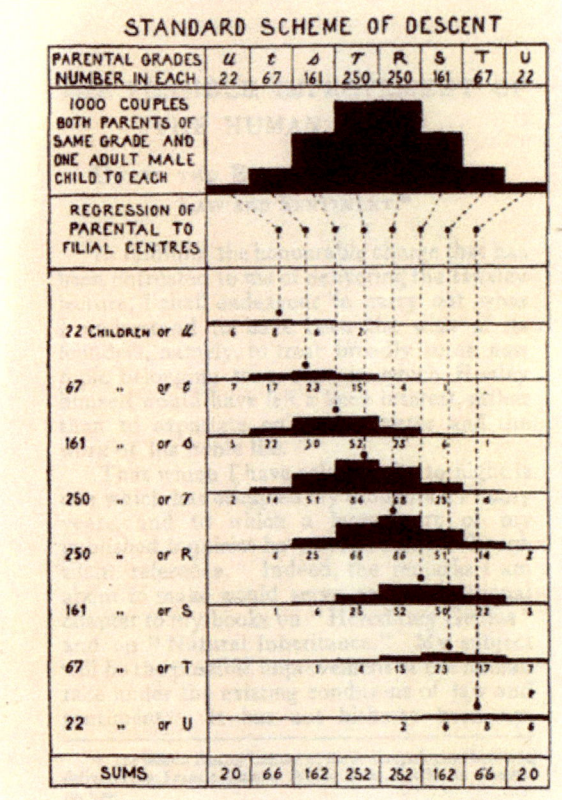

Figure 6. Regression to the mean

I realise I have perhaps concentrated too much on his contributions to science and not enough on his eccentricities:
- his calculation, whilst admiring a picture, that it contained 48,000 brush strokes,
- his nationwide survey of female allure, which led him to conclude that Aberdeen had the ugliest girls in Britain
- his invention of underwater spectacles for reading in the bath which led to a near drowning experience and another mental breakdown.

Galton was aware of his foibles and could laugh at himself, but he also knew that the path between genius and madness was a narrow one. He had walked the ground on both sides.

How does one summarise his career? No winner of the Royal Geographical Society's gold medal, of honorary degrees from both Oxford and Cambridge, of the Huxley Medal, the Darwin Medal and the Darwin-Wallace Medal and finally, in 1909, a knighthood should be overlooked, yet he remained the quintessential amateur, one of the last of a breed of Victorian polymaths. Although much of his scientific thinking was biased and opinionated, he nevertheless scored an amazing number of bullseyes. Trespassing into fields already trodden by others, he made lasting contributions to meteorology, geography, statistics, psychology, audiology and criminology. I have left eugenics to the last. Those of whom he approved should be encouraged to marry and breed – so far so good. Idiots and the unsalvageable should be sterilised, compulsorily if necessary. Charity in the form of scholarships was acceptable, but not charity to those less well endowed. The bell curve was to be shifted to the right by a process of natural attrition, assisted by stern indifference. Towards the end of his life he started to write a novel. Called *"Kantsaywhere"*. It is a description of a state where full eugenic principles are applied. It is so chillingly dystopic that Galton failed to finish it and asked for it to be destroyed after his death. It exists only in a heavily redacted manuscript which puts even *"Brave New World"* into the shade. Perhaps we should leave the last word to one of his disciples:

"At last there is a translation of the work of this great Englishman! He says all that I feel about the necessity to weed out the impure strains of race .... and leave the pure gold of the Nordic peoples"
That, of course was Heinrich Himmler.

The first Medical Missionary to India

MICHAEL WHITFIELD
Presented December 2013

As a schoolboy I read a lot about the early missionaries and I suppose my heroes at that time were people such as David Livingstone who went to Africa, William Carey, to India and Mary Slessor to Nigeria. Most of these were evangelists, but there were also a significant number of doctors, who, whilst seeking to spread the Gospel, also saw the need to use their medical skills. Many of these missionaries and members of their families lost their lives as they lived in very inclement climates. Nowadays, mission work still goes on but many question this approach and many countries don't welcome people from the UK who try to convert their people to the Christian faith.

Some of you will know of my particular interest in India and about three years ago, whilst visiting Calcutta, I was taken by a friend, to Serampore (about 10 miles along the river from Calcutta). This was the site where William Carey, whom I had always assumed was the first UK missionary, worked translating the bible and eventually had converts to Christianity.

The modern missionary movement has lasted over two hundred years and I want to tell you about someone who preceded Carey about whom I had never heard until about a year ago. He was a doctor who had been born in Fairford, Gloucestershire in 1757.

John Thomas was the second son of the village baker and miller. His father was a deacon in the small Baptist church in the village and John was said to have been a somewhat precocious lad who said he wanted to become a preacher even at the age of five. His mother died when he was eleven and this may have resulted in some adolescent misbehaviour as he was said to have avoided school and spent a lot of time indulging in shooting and fishing. He ran away from home, but somehow managed to get trained in medicine at the Westminster Hospital, London and obtained his Membership of the College of Surgeons.

After qualifying he became assistant surgeon on a naval ship, but after a serious feverish illness was admitted to the Haslar Naval Hospital, unconscious. After recovering he set up as a surgeon and apothecary in Great Newport Street in London. He married well, to a cousin of a Northamptonshire Squire in 1781, but things did not go well for this young doctor. He was no businessman and got himself into debt and was briefly imprisoned for this. There is some evidence of mental instability in that he was excitable and yet subject to despondent gloom. A friend helped him obtain a post as a ship's surgeon on an East India Company ship sailing to India.

He seemed to have had a successful voyage and managed to successfully treat many on his ship and those on other ships when in harbour in Calcutta. Whilst there he visited the city and attempted to seek out Christians but was unsuccessful in this. He even put a notice in the local paper asking whether anyone shared his idea of sharing the knowledge of Christ with the Bengalis.

'Religious Society

A plan is now forming for the more effectually spreading the knowledge of Jesus Christ, and the glorious gospel, in and about Bengal. Any serious persons, of any denomination, rich or poor, high or low, who would heartily approve of, or join in, or gladly

forward such an undertaking, are hereby invited to give a small testimony of their inclination, that they may enjoy the satisfaction of forming a communion the most useful, the most comfortable, and the most exalted in the world.
   Contact ABC through the editor'.

He didn't get any satisfactory reply to this.

He returned to the UK where he again attempted to get back into practice in London, in Great Portland Street (then on the northern extreme of the city) but again without much financial success. He became much more active in the local Baptist churches, became baptised and even considered becoming a pastor to a small church in Hertfordshire. His debts, though caught up with him and he decided to sail again to Calcutta on the same ship as before in 1786.

During this visit to Calcutta he met up with Charles Grant, a Scottish businessman, who was a senior officer of the East India Company. Grant held similar evangelical views to Thomas and had for some time, wanted to convert the Hindus and Moslems to Christianity. The East India Company, however, wanted none of this, as clearly this might interfere with their trading. Thomas convinced Grant of his abilities and was asked to consider becoming a missionary but was concerned about his ability to learn the language and also about having left his wife back in London.

Grant persuaded Thomas to move to Malda – a settlement three hundred miles north of Calcutta, where Grant's friend George Udny had a house. Thomas described a typical day in 1787:

'At 6 o'clock there is a large bell rung, which calls the party to a chapel in the house... we then breakfast and find it half past seven; I allot the following hours till ten for sweet meditation, reading and prayer; but it is very short. From ten till two I allot for the study of Bengali; rise from dinner before four; then sleep (according to the

custom of the country), read, ride out in a carriage (for we have no less than 7 carriages) in the cool of the evening, and rise from the tea table at about half past seven. Allow till nine for the study of the language and till ten for private devotion, at which hour we all meet again.'

One of the other East India company employees, living at Malda wrote a letter home at the end 1787 saying:

'God has been pleased to add another man, Dr Thomas, to our little family, and everyone of us has great reason for thankfulness for such a gracious providence. He was surgeon of the Oxford Indiaman, but a desire of becoming serviceable to the souls of the heathen here induced him to leave his post on board ship, and to remain in the country. He has been blessed with great gifts for preaching and praying, and gives us a regular discourse, extempore, twice every Sunday and short exhortations frequently on other occasions. He is now busy learning the Bengal language, and being of a conciliating temper, he may very probably, through the blessing of God, become serviceable to the natives as well as us'.

Unfortunately, this optimistic state of affairs did not last as Thomas ran into many problems. First, he antagonised Charles Grant, who was financing him. Thomas tried to persuade some of his colleagues in Malda to the Baptist persuasion. He tried to get his early translation of part of the New Testament published but Grant did not believe (with much justification) that Thomas had had time to master the language and Thomas did not take kindly to being restrained in this way. Eventually he was persuaded to move from Malda and Grant severed his connection with him.

Thomas continued to preach to the Bengalis and as he appeared to be well accepted by them, he decided to return to England, to try to find a fellow labourer and get financial support and to return with a printing press. He left India in 1792.

Meanwhile in England a group of Baptist preachers met together at Kettering, Northamptonshire in October 1792 and decided to set up a Society for Propagating the Gospel among the Heathen. This included a Northamptonshire Baptist minister called William Carey. Some of the members of the committee had heard of Thomas's wish to return to India and invited Thomas to attend a meeting of the committee and at the meeting Carey agreed to return with Thomas the next spring.

They attempted to get permission from the East India

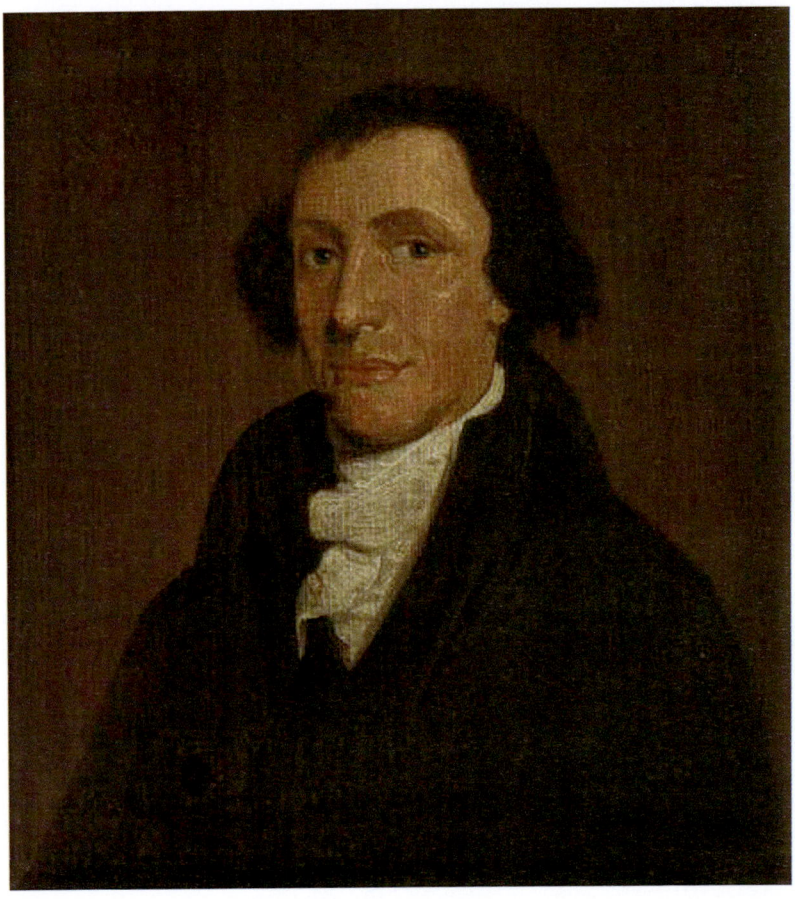

Figure 1. John Thomas

Company to return to Calcutta, but, unfortunately Charles Grant had now been appointed a Director of the Company and had moved to London. He refused to give that permission especially as Thomas was involved.

Nevertheless Thomas and Carey together with their wives and children eventually set sail in a Danish ship for India, Dorothy Carey just having given birth to her fourth child. They all arrived at Calcutta in November 1793. During the voyage Thomas started teaching Carey Bengali and on arrival they immediately ran into financial problems as Thomas attempted to run a medical practice and ran into further debt.

Things became very desperate for the two families and Carey and his family ended up living in very poor circumstances to the south of Calcutta.

It was about this time that George Udny entered the story again as his brother and wife, who were visiting, drowned tragically in a boating accident in Calcutta. Thomas heard about this tragedy wrote a letter of condolence to George Udny and was invited to visit Malda again. Udny invited Thomas and Carey to act as managers of two indigo factories he had in the neighbourhood. Each of these, which were twenty miles apart, provided work and, more importantly income for the two men. Another positive thing about these jobs was that indigo factories only required about three months intensive work each year, so both men were able to continue with their language lessons and the translation work. They were also not dependent on the Baptists in the UK finding money for the two missionary families.

After Carey suffered an attack of malaria, Udny sent both men up river to Bhutan for convalescence and they considered setting up mission there, but decided against it.

In 1795 Thomas sent a long letter home:

' We seldom have less than 800 people, servants, labourers and workmen, under our eye, at the two places, besides the natives who

plant the indigo, which are about 1000 more...'
He then described dinner (which was just ready) ....
'A boiled fowl, a glass of Madeira, with good bread and water'.
He wrote about his travels by river between the two factories:
'This moment six watermen are pulling us up the stream by a rope fastened to the top of the mast. One is picking fish for their dinner, one is posted to fend the boat occasionally from the banks, one steering and the rest are waiting for their turn on the rope. Betsey (Thomas's daughter) is laid on a sofa behind me fast asleep. Mrs T. is winding cotton before me'
Thomas was frequently called upon for his medical skills and several sheds were put up to shelter some of his patients – probably the first mission hospital!
In 1795 Dorothy Carey, William's wife, was causing both men major problems. Carey wrote home that his wife was looked upon as insane by both the natives and Europeans. Thomas wrote to the Chair of the Baptist Committee that:
'Do you know she has taken into her head that Carey is a great whoremonger; her jealousy burns like fire inquenchable; and this horrible idea has night and day filled her heart from about ten months past, so that if he goes out of his door by day or night she follows him: and declares in the most solemn manner that she has catched him with his servants, with his friends, with Mrs Thomas and that he is guilty every day and every night; I have listened to all her words and for a long time was in doubt whether she was actually possessed by a devil or insane. But by reading Dr Arnold on Notional Insanity I concluded the latter to be the case.'
Apparently on one occasion she held up a knife and said 'Curse you and I could cut your throat'.
After a year or so more, the indigo business was not doing very well and Thomas lost his job. Carey decided to move to Serampore near the Danish settlement and Thomas joined him there.
In 1799 a Bengali man arrived at Serampore with a dislocated

shoulder and Thomas was able to reduce this. At the same time he convinced the man called Krishna Pal to become a Christian. And in 1800 this man was baptised in the river by Carey – their first convert after many years in India. Thomas was so excited about this event that he went mad and needed to be confined. One description of the event was as follows:

'When Carey led Krishna and his own son Felix down into the water of baptism the ravings of Thomas in the schoolhouse on the one side, and of Mrs Carey on the other, mingled with the strains of the Bengali hymn of praise'.

Thomas was admitted to the Calcutta hospital for lunatics where he was confined for three weeks. He was then discharged to a friend and lived some miles north of Malda where he continued his work for about another year before dying of high fever and palpitations at the age of 44. His wife died the next year in Calcutta and his daughter returned to Fairford in Gloucestershire, where she married the local Baptist minister.

Thomas was always at the extreme of exultation or despondency but his short life was crucial in the development of Christianity in India. He exhibited many of the signs of bipolar disease but managed to achieve much in his young life.

A History of ECT
Dr Peter Carpenter
Presented September 2013

When electro convulsive therapy (ECT) was developed it was one of the safest and most effective treatments in psychiatry. In the 19th century the main treatment provided in psychiatry was good food to deal with the effects of malnutrition with opium and cathartics to sedate and quieten. Bromide arrived in 1892 to provide tranquilization and anti-epilepsy control, soon to be improved with the introduction of phenobarbitone in 1902.

Syphilis was treated with Mercury, with all its side effects. The novel effective physical therapy for Syphilis was Malarial Fever therapy started in 1917 by Wagner-Jauregg.

Malaria Fever therapy was seen as helping in some case of schizophrenia and mood disorder and was still in use in Glenside after the war. However the next advance was Insulin Coma therapy. This was developed by Manfred Sakel, who was a Jew born in Vienna how moved to work in Budapest. This was developed in 1924 but introduced more widely in 1934. It spread rapidly to the States in 1935, the United Kingdom in 1938 and was still in use in the States in the 1970's. It was dangerous - it was the injection of insulin to produce a coma - and usually a seizure. It had a death rate, but produced 50 - 80% remission in patients with schizophrenia.

Ladislaus Meduna, or Von Meduna as he called himself to cover up his Jewish ancestry, was a psychiatrist working in Budapest where he worked in a brain research with Scaffer who felt that Schizophrenia is inborn and untreatable. During the late 1920s he became interested in the apparent incompatibility of Epilepsy with Schizophrenia - their brain histology was different and in clinical practice saw very few patients with both schizophrenia and epilepsy. He later found that in the state asylum they did occur together, but when patients with epilepsy developed schizophrenia their epilepsy often improved.

He decided to try treating schizophrenia with seizures. His means of inducing seizures was to inject camphor, which takes some time to induce the seizure. His first patient was a man with catatonic schizophrenia, who had not moved for four years. He was first injected on 23 January 1934 and took 45 minutes to have a seizure. Meduna collapsed due to the tension after the patient recovered. Two days after the 5th injection the patient got up, walked and asked for breakfast. He could not believe he had been in hospital for four years but could recall what had been said around him when in his coma. He relapsed and had a further injection, when he recovered and met his wife. He relapsed again and was injected again - he recovered and escaped from hospital, to visit his wife, who he found had a lover, and beat the lover up. He was judged recovered.

The first five patients given Camphor all recovered. Meduna moved to using Metrazol as a faster way to induce seizures. In 1937 he published a case series of 110 patients, claiming 80% remission, with a much lower complication rate than Insulin Coma Therapy.

Meduna always saw Metrazol as a stop gap for inducing seizures. It took several minutes of arousal before the seizure occurred and further seizures could happen later in the same day. It was Ugo Cerletti who used Electricity to induce the seizures. Cerletti was born near Venice in 1877 and worked through clinics in Italy to become professor in Genoa in 1928 and in Rome in 1935. In 1936 he looked at insulin coma therapy and Metrazol therapy in

Budapest and researched using electricity to induce seizures in dogs. His initial work was unsuccessful and he was always aware of the image of electricity as a means of execution.

His first human patient was Enrico who he gave a shock to on 11 April 1938. The shocks were too weak to cause a seizure. He tried it on a woman and then again on Enrico, with a higher voltage of 92 volts and on 20 April 1938 induced his first seizure lasting ten minutes. After a course of seven to eight seizures Enrico was writing letters. Enrico was presented to the Royal Academy of Rome on the 28 May when Cerletti gave him ECT on stage. Cerletti and his assistant Bini seem to have minimised the side effects and became showmen like Walter Freeman - in his hospital trumpets signalled when he was giving ECT for doctors to assemble and watch.

In 1938 a company was contracted to make the machines according to Bini's design. A second assistant Kalinowsky, a german psychiatrist with Jewish heritage escaped Germany to work with them, but then as the war loomed travelled across Europe to England and then the States, spreading the news of ECT, calling it the Cerletti-Bini treatment - to the annoyance of Cerletti. By 1940 it was recognised that ECT worked best for severe depression.

Though the States was a country dominated by psychoanalytical therapy, ECT was well supported and psychiatrists recognised that ECT worked when psychotherapy did not. It was cheap and effective, however in the United States it got a reputation in the state asylums as a method of control as the attendants selected who was given it.

In England it was established in 1939, championed by Michael Shepherd in the Maudsley and Max Hamilton in Leeds. At the Burden Clinic Professor Golla had Grey Walter make a machine and they tested it on sheep, before using it on five patients and publishing this with Dr Fleming (of Barnwood house, Gloucester). The Monica Britton Museum had one of the first machines used at the Burden Clinic, and it is now in the Science Museum. Glenside Museum has a slightly later one in its diorama, which is the same one seen in a film on ECT of the time.

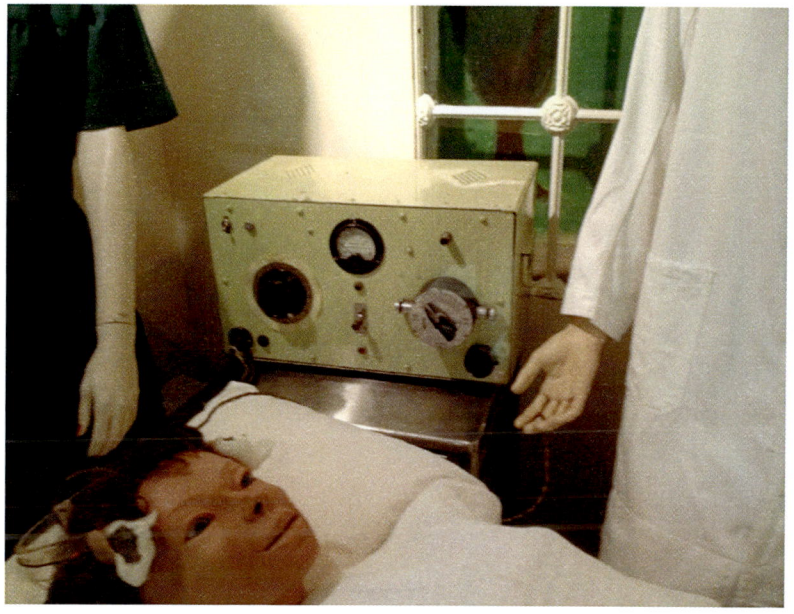

The Diorama at Glenside Museum showing a 1948 ECT machine.

ECT became popular as is was as effective as Insulin Coma Therapy and Metrazol Therapy but was much safer and easier to administer. Antidepressants were first developed in 1957 but ECT remained the more effective.

In its unmodified form there was a risk of fractures, particularly of the spine, which was reduced dramatically by arching the back over a sandbag. Anaesthetic was introduced in the 1950s but many argued that ECT was not as effective if the seizure was suppressed. There were also complaints of memory loss. How much this was due to the anaesthetic or the shock was not clear. However there was a lot of research done - indeed ECT can claim to be the most researched treatment in medicine to no clear conclusion. However Neville Lancaster with Steinert and Frost in Chester researched and used unilateral ECT where the electrodes were not placed on both temples but both on the non-dominant side of the brain, one behind the other. This seemed to produce less memory problems but many felt it was not as effective.

Though the Psychiatrists felt ECT was very useful and effective, popular resistance to it grew in as part of the anti-psychiatry movement of the 1960's. It was shown in Snake Pit in 1948 and One Flew over the Cuckoo's Nest in 1975, both as tortures and I have read claims that no film showing ECT has yet shown it used with anaesthetic, It is always shown in its most dramatic form - *'They are going to fry your brains'*.

The use of ECT has diminished dramatically to the point that now in Avon there is only one suite and many days no one receiving it. Newer medications have reduced the need but cynically one wonders what role the Pharma companies had in the anti-ECT movement. The Mental Health Act now requires quite a complex certification process for it to be given.

However in the Third World it remains the cheapest physical treatment available, when given without anaesthetic and still has a reputation as an agent of control. There are trials to replace ECT with Transcranial Magnetic Therapy and Deep Brain Stimulation but these have yet to prove either as simple to give or as effective.

Abstract
Fin-de-siècle: male hysteria

Tom Nutting,
Medical Student
PRESENTED 17.3.2014

This essay aims to delineate a history of hysteria with a particular interest in the emergence of a male variant of the diagnosis. As such, the main point of focus is neurologist Jean-Martin Charcot's model of the disease in fin-de-siècle Paris, which affected both men and women. I consider some of the feminist interpretations of this model of hysteria and ask if it can still be regarded as enforcing traditional gender roles. I conclude that whilst Charcot was driven to push a male model of the disorder to ensure occupational success, he modulated this so that it did little to challenge accepted notions of gender; like his contemporaries, Charcot was not exempt from the political and psychological pressures that cultivated resistance to a truly universal model of hysteria. I apply Jewson's 'medical cosmologies' to this history, arguing this can highlight how the social structure of medicine perpetuated Charcot's model of hysteria. Finally, I suggest two possible reasons for the under-discussion of male hysteria in historical studies: that they have been largely dominated by feminist criticism, and that male hysteria could only be discussed fully at the next fin-de-siècle after certain sociocultural developments of the twentieth century.

Edith and Florence Stoney, X-ray pioneers

Francis Duck MBE, PhD DSc
3 Evelyn Road Bath BA1 3QF
f.duck@bath.ac.uk
Presented 16.6.2014

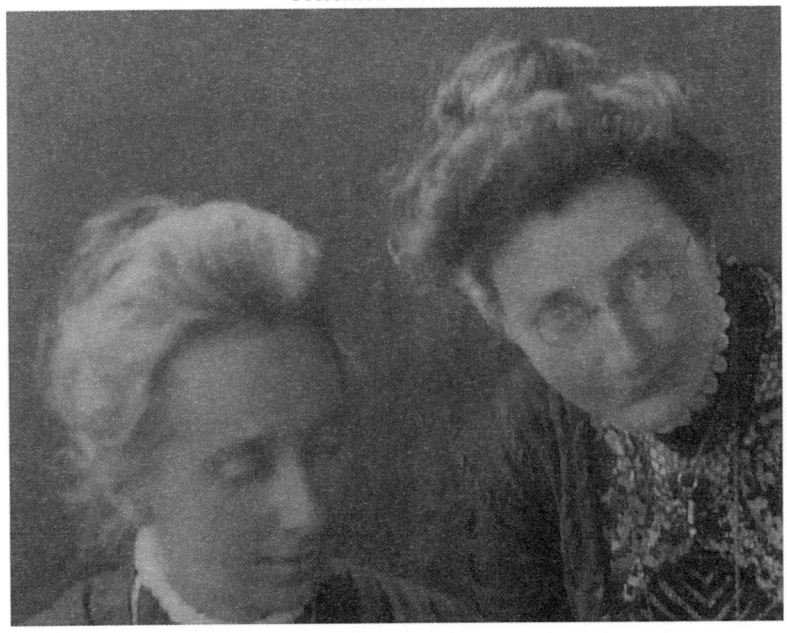

Figure 1 Edith (L) and Florence (R) Stoney. c. 1910.
Newnham College Archive.

Edith Anne Stoney (1869-1938) and Florence Ada Stoney (1870 – 1932) (Figure 1) were born in Dublin into a scientific family. Their father, G. Johnstone Stoney FRS, an eminent physicist, coined the term 'electron' in 1891 as the "fundamental unit quantity of electricity", four years before its experimental demonstration by J J Thomson. Their engineer uncle Bindon Blood Stoney, their engineer brother Gerald and their physicist cousin, George FitzGerald, were all awarded FRS [1].

The girls were educated privately and then at the Royal College for Science of Ireland. Edith gained a scholarship to Newnham College, Cambridge, where she achieved a First in the Part I Maths Tripos examination in 1893. She was later awarded MA from Trinity College Dublin, after they accepted women in 1904. After graduation she carried our some difficult calculations on marine turbine engines and searchlight design for Sir Charles Parsons, and then took a mathematics teaching post at Cheltenham Ladies' College.

By this time, Florence had started training at the London School of Medicine for Women (LSMW) where she obtained her MD in 1898. The following year Edith moved back to London when she was appointed as physics lecturer at the LSMW [2] (Figure 2).

Florence was working as an anatomy demonstrator at LSMW and as a clinical assistant in ENT at the Royal Free Hospital. In 1901 she

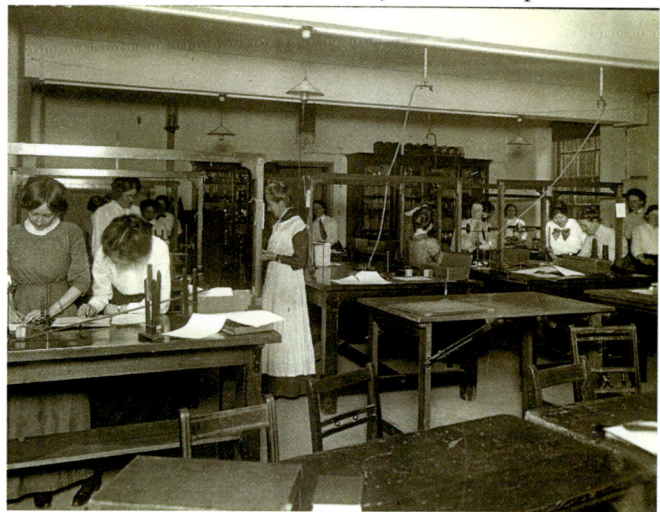

Figure 2. Edith Stoney teaching in her physics laboratory at the London (Royal Free) School of Medicine for Women. c. 1910. Royal Free Archives, London Metropolitan Archives.

was also appointed to the post of medical electrician. The two sisters set about selecting, purchasing and installing x-ray equipment and, the following April, a new x-ray service was opened [3].

Florence soon moved to the New Hospital for Women to become the head of the electrical department, and in 1906 set up in practice in Harley Street. She developed her skills and knowledge in radiology and electrotherapy. In particular she started to use x-rays to treat uterine fibroids and ophthalmic goitre [4]. In 1914 she travelled in America, visiting a number of radiological centres to learn of best practice there [5]. She returned with one of the new Coolidge tubes and became one of the very first to start using this technological breakthrough in Britain.

The two women were also actively involved in the women's movement. As the first treasurer of the Federation of Women Graduates, Edith pressed for women to be permitted to practice law, to take senior positions in prison management and, later, receive training to fill jobs vacated by men during the war [6].

Britain declared war on Germany on 4 August 1914. The same day, Florence and Edith offered their services to the British Red Cross at the War office in London to provide a radiological service to support the troops in Europe. Their offer was refused, because they were women. Undaunted, Florence became the medical lead of an all-women unit funded by the Women's Imperial Service League. They established a hospital in Antwerp in September, but were quickly in retreat from the German advance. They then set up in Cherbourg, accepting casualties brought in by sea. Edith organised supplies from London where she also served on the League's committee [7]. Florence returned to London in March 1915, her arrival coinciding with Edith's resignation from the LSMW.

Florence was then appointed as head of radiology at the 1000-bed Fulham Military Hospital, one of the first women to be accepted by the War Office. After the war she would be awarded the OBE for her services there. Edith contacted the Scottish Women's Hospitals

(SWH), an organisation formed in 1914 to give medical support in the field of battle, financed by the women's suffrage movement. In June 1915 she set off to Europe, and would be away for most of the next four years. The SWH had gained agreement to set up a new 250-bed tented hospital at Troyes [8]. It was Edith's task to plan and operate the x-ray facilities, for which her only assistant in this otherwise all-female unit was George Mallett, a young engineer who had been trained by her sister. Following her sister's lead, she established methods for the geometric localization of bullets and shrapnel and introduced the use of x-rays in the diagnosis of gas gangrene, interstitial gas being a mandate for immediate amputation to give any chance of survival [9] (Figures 3 and 4).

These summer months in northern France acclimatized Edith to the challenge of front-line military radiography, with its traumatically injured soldiers and difficult working conditions. In September, they were assigned to the Corps Expéditionnaire d'Orient, and set off for Serbia. Edith was concerned about the availability

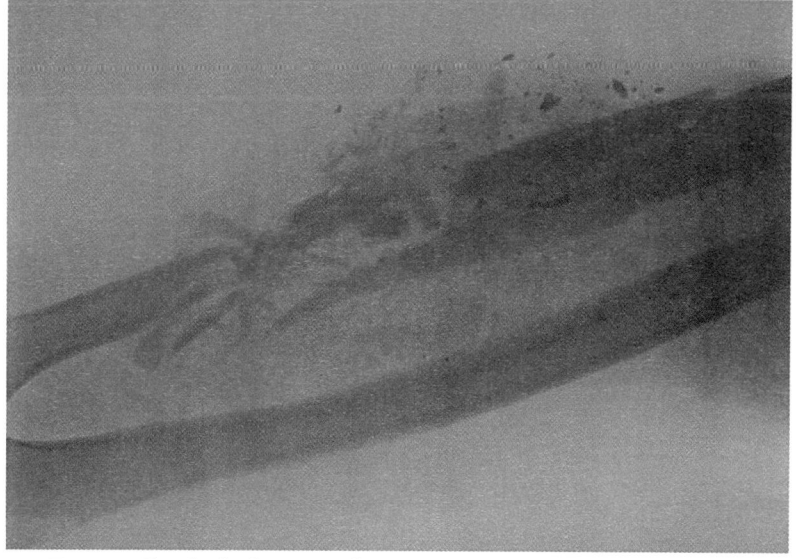

Figure 3 Cloudy shadow on radiograph, indicative of gas gangrene. [9]

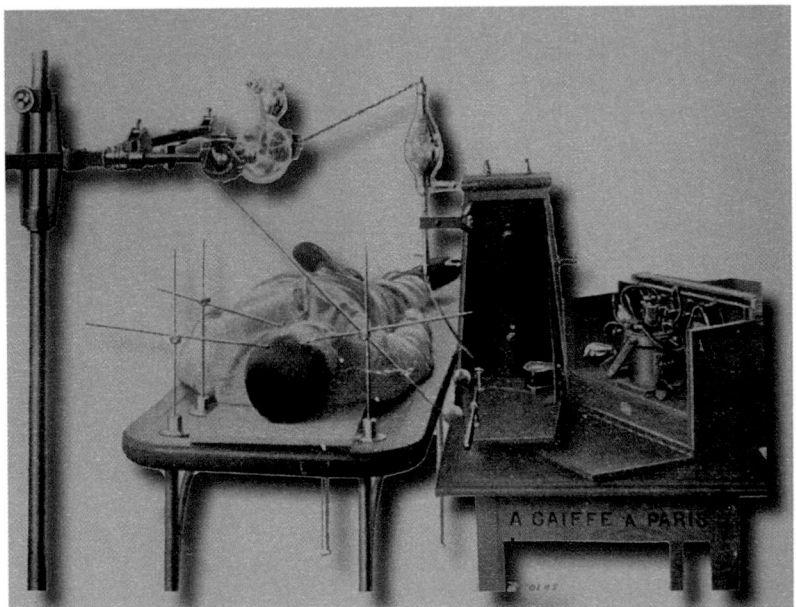

Figure 4 One of the complex methods for the location of foreign bodies introduced during WWI.

of electricity where they were going and, when her request for a generator was turned down, she bought one herself during a lightning visit to Paris.

By early November the unit had reached Ghevgheli in Serbia where they set up in an unused silk factory. The conditions were cold and difficult but Edith reported that the view was lovely and the air was bracing. However, they were on the southern flank of a loosing battle for Serbia against the Bulgarian forces. By December 6th they were back in Salonica, evacuated down the single-track railway, the factory burnt and blown up behind them [10].

Edith spent most of 1916 running the x-ray service in the camp in Salonica, ably assisted by Mallett, and working closely with a Parisian physicist, Charles Géneau, who was running an equivalent service in the neighbouring French hospital. They were in a war zone still, with air raids once or twice a week. Having set up the electricity supply, Edith established an electrotherapy department, including electrical massage, ionisation therapy, high-frequency heating, electrical baths and heat lamps. But not all went smoothly. When the x-ray van arrived she found that it had insufficient clearance for the rough roads, and vibration from the dynamo caused blurring of the x-ray images (Figure 5).

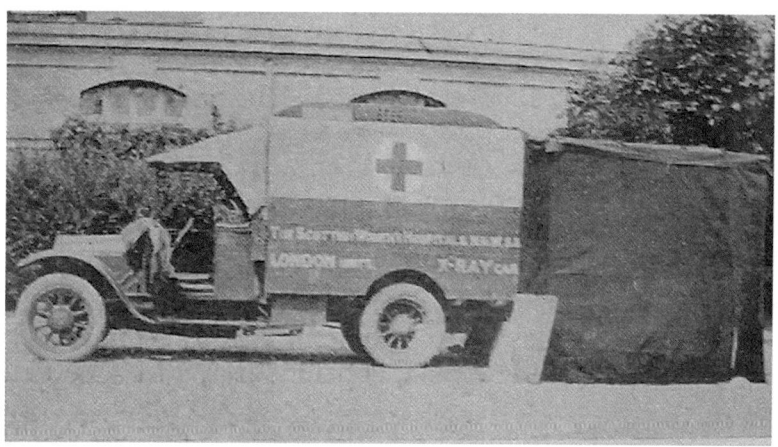

Figure 5. The x-ray van of the London Unit of the Scottish Women's Hospitals, based at Royaumont, France. [16] . *Wellcome Library, London.*

The summer months were hot and difficult, with staff illnesses and patients with malaria and dysentery. Finally, in October 1917, she returned to northern France to lead the X-ray departments at the SWH hospitals at Royaumont and Villers-Cotterêts.

In March 1918, she once more had to supervise a camp closure and retreat, when Villers-Cotterêts was overrun by the advancing front. During the final months of the war the fighting intensified and there was a huge increase in workload. In the month of June 1918 alone the x-ray workload peaked at over 1300, partly resulting from an increased use of fluoroscopy (Figure 6). This arose partly from the immediateness of the diagnosis and partly from concern about the escalating cost of film. However, it also resulted in an increased incidence of radiation burns to Edith's staff, two of whom had to take sick leave to recover.

From London, Florence recognised the extreme strain her sister was under. She wrote.. " *We may indeed be proud of them all but I fear there will be a heavy aftermath to pay for the great overwork they are undergoing. Here, in London, we think we are busy, but it is a backwater compared to Royaumont,"* adding *"She is not at all well – it is the price she has to pay for the help she has given during the war. Few people realise what the constant strain of x-ray work … If she had been in the army she would have had a pension."* [11]

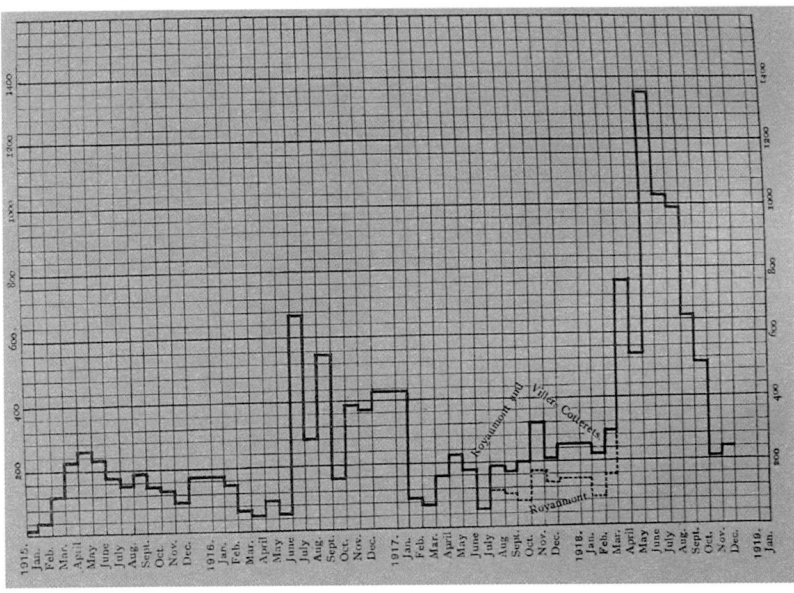

Figure 6 Edith Stoney's statistical report showing the large increase in x-ray studies in the summer of 1918 at Royaumont and Villers-Cotterêts. [8] *380. Wellcome Library, London.*

The last point was important. Edith needed work at the end of the war, but met considerable resistance when she tried to capitalize on her radiological skills, because she was not medically qualified and also partly because she was a woman [12]. After the war ended she went back to academic physics, teaching at King's College for Women, before retiring in 1925.

Florence's health was suffering by the end of the war, and she moved to Bournemouth where she practiced radiology part-time. Edith joined her after her retirement, and they travelled together, including trips to India and South Africa, where Florence studied the association between UV exposure, vitamin D and skeletal development. Following Florence's early death from vertebral cancer in 1932, Edith continued to travel. She represented the British Federation for University Women in Australia, and set up a travel bursary for scientific women graduates, which she supported by a further £3000 legacy when she died in 1938.

Obituaries recognised the contributions that both women had made to radiology and to the cause of women's education [13,14,15]. They were highly intelligent, tough and single-minded women. They both demonstrated high organizational skills in challenging circumstances. They showed considerable bravery and resourcefulness in the face of extreme danger, and imagination in contributing to clinical care under the most difficult conditions of war. In the history of early years of radiology and of medical physics, Edith and Florence Stoney stand out as two of the most able pioneers.

REFERENCES

1) Jean M Guy. Edith (1869-1938) and Florence (1870-1932) Stoney, two Irish sisters and their contribution to radiology during Word War I. J Med Biog 2013;21:100-107.
2) Council minutes of the London (Royal Free) School of Medicine for Women. Archives of the Royal Free Hospital. London Metropolitan Archives
3) Florence A Stoney. Rœntgen Rays at the Royal Free. London School of Medicine for Women Magazine. Jan 1903. 133-135.
4) Florence Ada Stoney. ON then results of treating exophthalmic goitre with X-rays. Archiv Roentgen Ray 1913;17:320-322.
5) Florence A Stoney. X-ray notes from the United States. Archiv Roentgen Ray October 1914:19:181-184.
6) Federation of University Women. Executive Committee Minutes 1909-1916. The Women's Library archive at the LSE. 5BFW/02/01.
7) Barbara MacLaren. Miss Edith Stoney and Dr Florence Stoney. Women of the War. London. Hodder & Stoughton. 1917. 41-46.
8) Eva Shaw McLaren. A History of the Scottish Women's Hospitals. London, Hodder & Stoughton. 1919.
9) Agnes Saville. X-ray apparatus in gas gangrene. Proc Roy Soc Med 1917;10:4-16.
10) Edith A Stoney. The Girton and Newnham Unit of the Scottish Women's Hospitals for Foreign Service, National Union of Women Suffrage Societies. Dec 12 1916. Newnham Letter Jan 1917. National Library of Scotland.
11) Eileen Crofton. The Women of Royaumont. A Scottish Women's Hospital on the Western Front. E Lothian, Tuckwell. 1997. 206.
12) Edith A Stoney to Sir James Mackenzie-Davidson. 7 July 1918. Mackenzie-Davidson papers. BIR Archives.
13) Florence Ada Stoney, O.B.E., M.D.(Lond.), D.M.R.E.(Camb). Br J Radiol 1932;5:853-858.
14) Edith Stoney, M.A. Lancet, July 9 1938. 108.
15) Miss Edith Stoney. Nature July 16, 1938. 103-104.
16) Mary H Frances Ivans. The part played by British medical women in the war. British Medicine in the War. BMA. 1917. 118.

Fetal Compression
and the Recognition of Congenital Deformation
1960-1981
PETER M. DUNN,

MA, MD, FRCP, FRCOG, FRCPCH
Emeritus Professor of Perinatal Medicine and Child Health
University of Bristol
(P.M.Dunn@bristol.ac.uk)

Presented June 2014

In August 1967 I was invited to speak at a perinatal conference organised by the University of Florida and held at the Plaza Hotel at Daytona Beach, home of many famous car races. I was delighted to find that the distinguished perinatal pathologist, Edith Potter, was also on the faculty[1] (Fig.1).

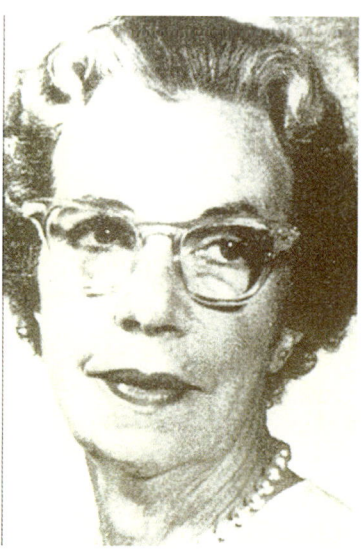

Fig.1 Dr. Edith Potter (1901-1993)

Born in 1901, she qualified in medicine at the University of Minneapolis in 1925. Nine years later in 1934, she was appointed first as instructor and then as professor of pathology at the Chicago Lying in Hospital. In 1952, on the basis of some 10,000 necropsies, she published her great work entitled 'The Pathology of the Fetus and Infant'[2]. Almost single handed Potter founded the new modern specialty of perinatal pathology. She died in 1993 at the age of 92.

Since her death in 1993, Edith Potter has been best remembered eponymously by the facial characteristics of infants born with bilateral renal agenesis[3]. She first described this facies in 1946 when she wrote:

'The peculiar facies of these infants seems to have no specific embryologic correlation with the renal anomaly. The face most characteristically exhibits an increased space between the eyes, a prominent fold which arises at the inner canthus and sweeps downward and laterally below the eyes, an unusual flattening of the nose, with excessive retraction of the chin ... and a moderate enlargement and decreased chondrification of the ears. The face gives a suggestion of premature senility and is sufficiently characteristic to warrant a diagnosis of co-existing renal aplasia when it is observed.' (Fig.2)

Edith Potter also observed that these babies usually had limb deformities such a club feet. In addition she recorded that they invariably had pulmonary hypoplasia . However, she was unable to explain the presence of this hypoplasia, pointing out that: 'There is no apparent relationship between the embryonic development of the lungs and the ureters and kidneys'. Although she recorded the probable association of the lack of amniotic fluid with bilateral renal agenesis, she did not relate the characteristic facies and associated deformities with prenatal fetal compression.

I remain especially grateful to Edith Potter in that the sight of a case of Potter's Syndrome in 1958 helped to stimulate my interest in prenatal fetal deformation. During the decade 1959-1968

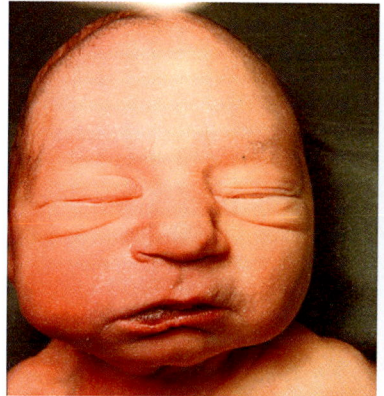 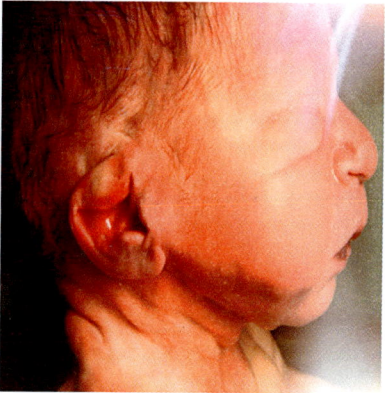

Fig.2a and 2b Potter's facies (front and side views).

I worked on a magnum opus entitled: *'The influence of the intrauterine environment on the causation of congenital postural deformities with special reference to congenital dislocation of the hip*[4]. When after three years of clinical research I began to study the literature on this subject, I found to my surprise that the notion that intrauterine constraint might lead to fetal deformation, though discounted in recent times, actually reached back to the days of Hippocrates[5]. It had never been discussed when I was a medical student and there was no mention of the idea in any of my medical textbooks. Furthermore I discovered that the idea had been vigorously advanced by Sir Denis Browne[6] (Fig.3) in 1934, though without achieving wide support. The orthopaedic world in particular dismissed and derided the idea that mechanical forces *inutero* might lead to fetal deformity.

The problem with the research of Sir Denis and others was that it was purely observational, unsupported by convincing scientific evidence.

However, my own observations were supported by such evidence in the form of epidemiological studies on a cohort of 6,756 consecutively newborn infants studied between 1960 and 1963. This enabled me to confirm my conclusions with the aid of 180 statistical analyses, some of them to be seen in Figure 4, which reveals that the main congenital postural deformities occur in association with each other.

Besides clinical and radiological studies I also made many pathological observations on this subject, courtesy of two pathologists, Dr. Hans Kohler in Birmingham, and Dr. Norman Brown in Bristol. All together I must have undertaken four or five hundred post-mortem examinations.

Returning to the subject of Potter's facies, perhaps the most

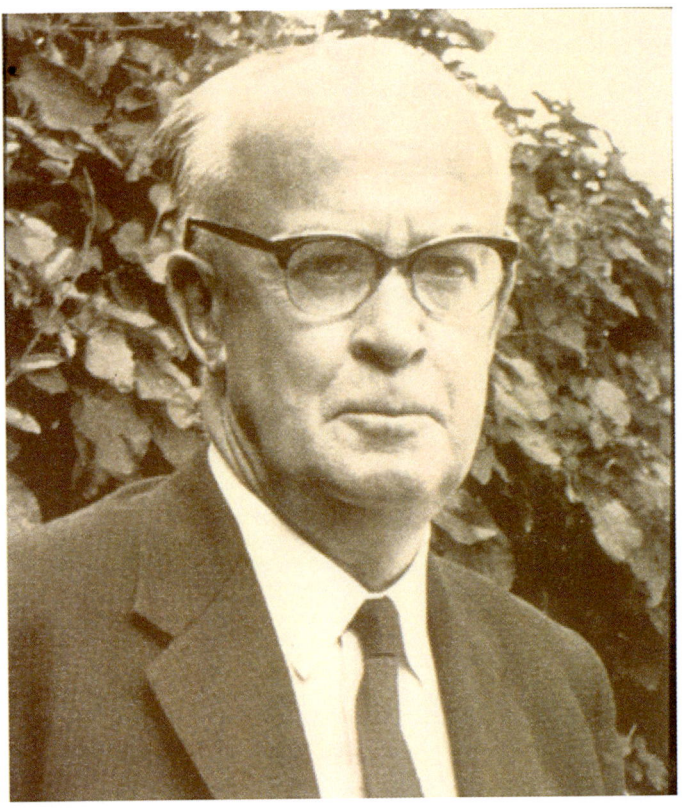

Fig.3 Sir Denis Browne (1892-1967)

fundamental observation I made in the early 1960s was of the highly significant association of Potters facies and other deformations with maternal oligohydramnios, whether due to bilateral renal malformation, whatever its nature – agenesis, polycystic kidneys, etc.-, or to prolonged leakage of amniotic fluid, or to the oligohydramnios associated with severe placental insufficiency. It was also highly significant that Potter's facies and limb deformities were not present when renal malformation was unilateral. However, they were present when there was severe urinary tract obstruction below the level of the bladder causing oligohydramnios. The critical factor was, of course, whether or not the fetus was able to pass

CONGENITAL POSTURAL DEFORMITIES	Facial def.	Plagioceph.	Mandib. asym.	Sternom. contr.	Scoliosis	C.D.H.	Talipes
Facial Deformities		S	S*	S	S*	S*	S*
Plagiocephaly	S		S*	S*	S*	S*	N
Mandibular asymmetry	S*	S*		S*	N	S*	S*
Sternomastoid contr.	S	S*	S*		S*	N	S*
Scoliosis - postural	S*	S*	N	S*		S*	S
Cong. Disloc. Hips	S*	S*	S*	N	S*		S*
Talipes	S*	N	S*	S*	S	S*	

N = not signif; S = P<0.05; S* = P<0.001

Fig.4 Statistical analysis of studies made during 1960-63 of the clinical association between certain congenital postural deformities (Dunn 1969(4)). Abbreviations: N: not significant; S: P<0.05; S*: P<0.001

urine *inutero*, and hence provide volume to the amniotic fluid.

Let me give two brief case histories in support of these observations:

- Case 1: Maternal oligohydramnios. Breech delivery at 37 weeks gestation. Male infant weighing 3.4Kg with Potter's facies and respiratory distress. Bilateral pneumothoraces drained. Died at 18 hours. Necropsy revealed urethral valves and dilation deformities of the bladder, ureters and kidneys. Pulmonary hypoplasia was present.
- Case 2: Maternal oligohydramnios secondary to premature rupture of the membranes and prolonged drainage of the amniotic fluid. Male infant with Potter's facies and postural deformities of the hands and feet (Fig.5). Kidneys and urinary tract normal.

In May 1968 my three volume thesis [4] was submitted to the University of Cambridge. Eight months were to pass before I was informed that it had been finally accepted for the degree of MD. Later, I heard that one of the assessors, a professor of orthopaedic surgery, had given it the thumbs down. Fortunately, the other assessor and an extra one called in to adjudicate had eventually given it their approval. Many papers based on my thesis followed[7-15] and in 1976 I was asked to summarise my findings in an edition of the British Medical Bulletin devoted to 'malformations'[16].

The distinguished Professor Tom McKeown of Birmingham, an expert in the etiology and epidemiology of congenital anomalies, was invited to review this edition of the bulletin. He commented: 'The significance of mechanical influences in the uterus on congenital postural deformities (reviewed by Dunn) is still an open question.'[17] Fortunately, not everyone was sceptical. In 1975 I was invited to take part in an International Conference on the Classification of Congenital Anomalies[18] at the National Institute of Health, Bethesda, under the Chairmanship of Dr. David Smith, author of the classic text, '*Recognisable Patterns of Human Malformation*'[19]. Both at that meeting and at a subsequent conference on the same subject in Baltimore chaired by Dr. Victor McKusick, I presented my ideas on the origin of congenital postural deformities. To my delight, they again received very strong support.

But what was my thesis?$_{(4,16)}$ In summary, it was that: *'Quite gentle forces, if persistently applied, might lead to deformation. That such deformation occurs much more readily in the presence of growth. That the fetus is particularly vulnerable to deformation because of its rapid rate of growth and relative plasticity. That prenatal deforming forces might be intrinsic or extrinsic in origin. That most fetuses were exposed*

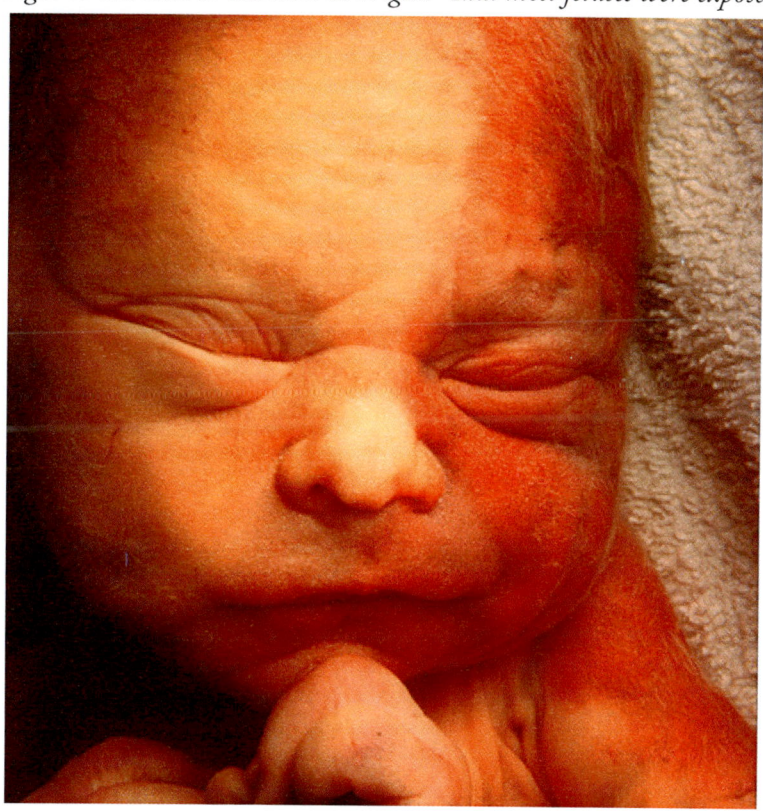

Fig. 5
Infant with classic Potter's facies and postural deformities secondary to oligohydramnios due to leakage of amniotic fluid.
Kidneys and urinary tract normal.

to extrinsic forces in the later weeks of pregnancy because of their increasing size and the diminishing volume of amniotic fluid. That at least 2% of infants exhibited postural deformities at birth though the great majority of these deformities either resolved spontaneously or responded to early postural correction.

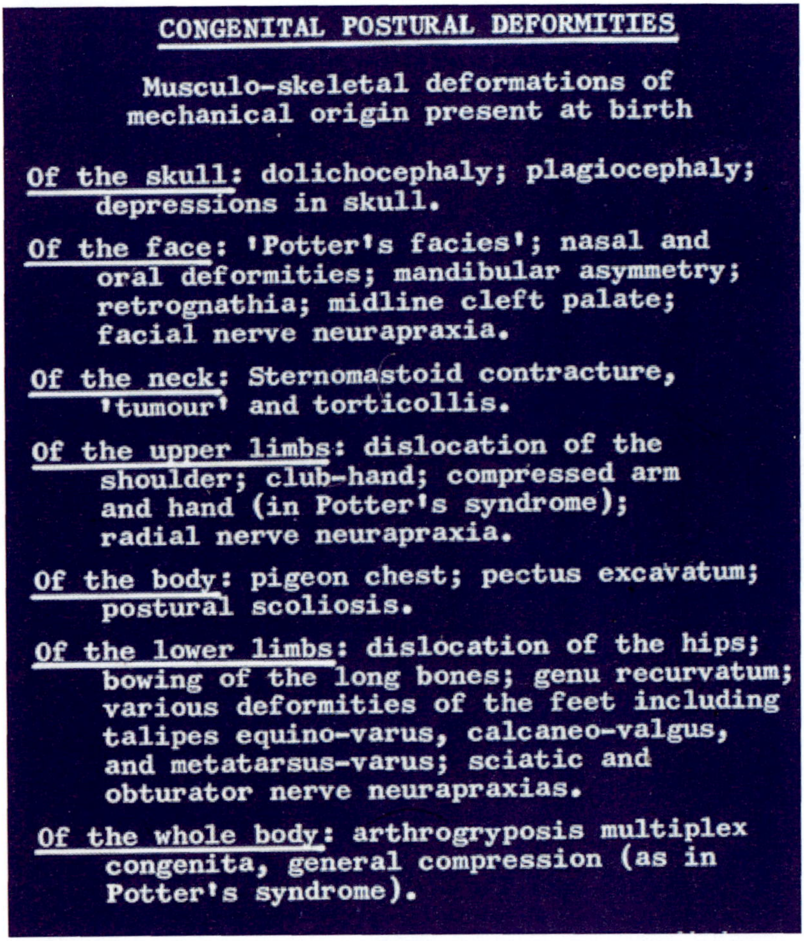

CONGENITAL POSTURAL DEFORMITIES

Musculo-skeletal deformations of mechanical origin present at birth

Of the skull: dolichocephaly; plagiocephaly; depressions in skull.

Of the face: 'Potter's facies'; nasal and oral deformities; mandibular asymmetry; retrognathia; midline cleft palate; facial nerve neurapraxia.

Of the neck: Sternomastoid contracture, 'tumour' and torticollis.

Of the upper limbs: dislocation of the shoulder; club-hand; compressed arm and hand (in Potter's syndrome); radial nerve neurapraxia.

Of the body: pigeon chest; pectus excavatum; postural scoliosis.

Of the lower limbs: dislocation of the hips; bowing of the long bones; genu recurvatum; various deformities of the feet including talipes equino-varus, calcaneo-valgus, and metatarsus-varus; sciatic and obturator nerve neurapraxias.

Of the whole body: arthrogryposis multiplex congenita, general compression (as in Potter's syndrome).

Fig.6
Congenital postural deformities in relation to the part of the body affected.

Figure 6 lists most of the main anomalies that I have termed the congential postural deformities in relation to the part of the body affected.

With the aid of epidemiological statistical analyses, it was possible to show that the various deformities seen in the last figure not only occurred in association with each other to a highly significant degree (Fig.4) but also occurred in association with the following pregnancy factors – first pregnancy, breech presentation, oligohydramnios, maternal hypertension and fetal growth retardation. Moreover, it was also possible to demonstrate how these pregnancy factors were related to each other and to the causation of fetal deformation[4,16] (Figs. 7 and 8).

The underlying significance of my thesis was that while

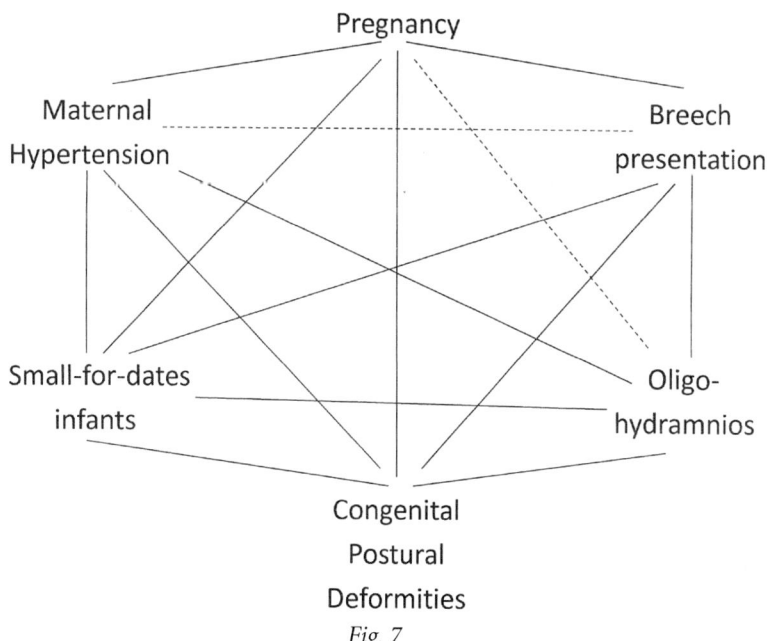

Fig. 7
Congenital postural deformation and certain pregnancy factors. (Dunn 1969[4]). Each unbroken line represents a statistically significant association, while the interrupted lines represent probable but unproven associations

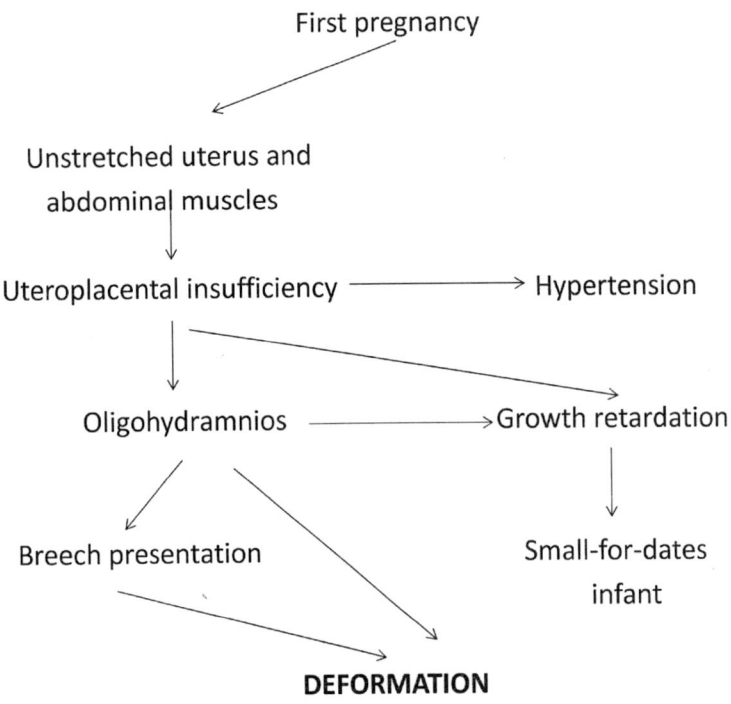

Fig. 8
Possible interrelation of some of the pregnancy associations with congenital postural deformation (Dunn 1969[4]).

malformations were defects arising during the period of organogenesis and were essentially teratological embyropathies, congenital deformations were defects arising after the embryonic period and were thus alterations in a previously normally formed part of the body. They were fetopathies. The importance of this distinction is absolutely fundamental to the understanding of their occurrence and management, as well as to the prognosis of these deformed infants involving some 2% of all newborn babies.

The support I received at those two conferences in the USA in 1975 was particularly helpful as at that time I had been engaged by the

World Health Organisation to help revise the 1967 eighth edition of the International Classification of Diseases$_{(20)}$. In chapter 14 of this revision, dealing with congenital anomalies, what I personally termed the postural deformations were all mixed up together with the malformations and were only related in the text to the anatomical part of the body involved. While it is not easy to bring about changes in the ICD, which is only revised about once a decade, I am happy to say that in ICD 9 (1979) my arguments in support of the separation of deformities from malformations were accepted with the result that the deformities were then segregated from the malformations with their own anatomic rubrics$_{(21)}$. As you may imagine, it gave me great satisfaction after having been told for many years that my ideas were ill-conceived. Later in the 1980s I was also invited to help to prepare the 10th revision of the International Classification of Diseases[22]. This provided another opportunity to further improve and bed down the deformation rubrics.

But there was yet another pleasure in store. In 1977 David Smith, doyen of dysmorphologists, rang me up and asked if he and his wife could come and stay with us in Bristol (Fig.9). It transpired that he had come over from Seattle, in order to read and photocopy my MD thesis[4] held in the Cambridge University Library.

Four years later in 1981 David Smith's secretary sent me, at his request, a copy of his new textbook, a companion to his earlier one, with the title: 'Recognisable Patterns of Human Deformation'[23]. Typical of the man, he had paid me generous credit in the preface. He wrote:

> *'It was in February, 1975, at an international meeting on Nomenclature for Birth Defects, that I first heard Peter Dunn, MD, of Bristol, England, give his impassioned plea for a clear distinction between defects due to mechanical constraint forces (deformation) as contrasted to those due to poor formation (malformation). His recommendation was accepted forthwith. Since that time, I*

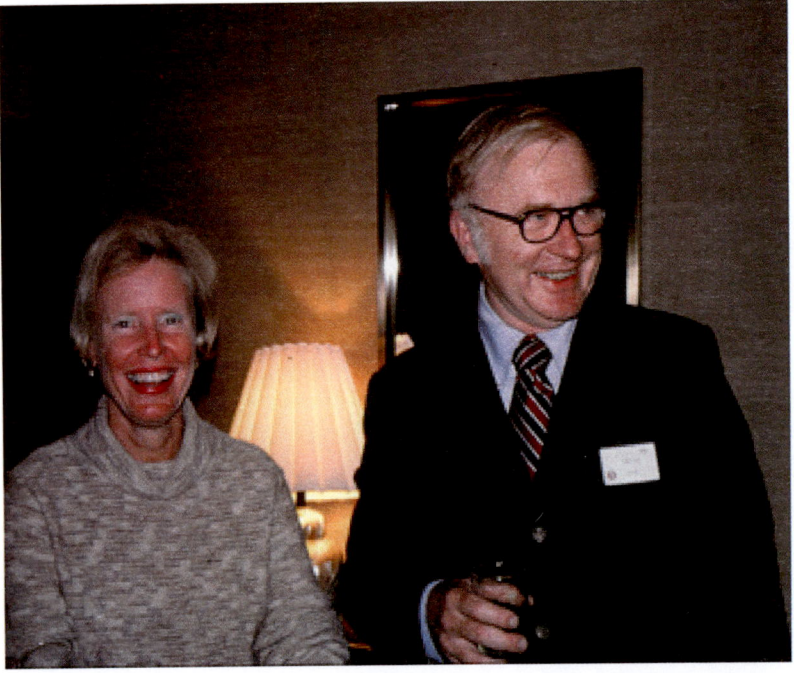

Fig.9   Prof. David Smith of Seattle with Mrs. Anne Smith (1977).

have been ever more impressed by the importance, relevance, and magnitude of this deformational category of birth defects. Hence, I acknowledge Peter Dunn as the individual who set me forth on the pathway that culminated in this book.'

I would, of course, have liked to have been able to thank David Smith both for the book and his kind acknowledgement but, sadly, I learnt that he had died one month before its publication
I fear as Shakespeare once said, *'All this comes too near the praising of myself'.* Please forgive me but over the whole 50 years since I first formulated my thesis on the nature of congenital postural deformation, this tribute by David Smith was the only public acknowledgement I have ever received. What had been considered

a misconceived idea, overnight had become an obvious truth. Meanwhile the author, previously considered to be a crank, has become a bore. Such is life!

REFERENCES

1. Dunn, P.M. Dr. Edith Potter (1901-1993) of Chicago: pioneer in perinatal pathology. Arch. Dis. Child. Neonatal Ed. 2007; 92, 419-420.
2. Potter, E.L. Pathology of the fetus and infant. Chicago: Year Book Medical Publ., 1952.
3. Potter, E.L. Facial characteristics of infants with bilateral renal agenesis. Amer. J. Obstet. Gynecol. 1946; 51, 885-8.
4. Dunn, P.M. The influence of the intrauterine environment in the causation of congenital postural deformities, with special reference to congenital dislocation of the hip. Vols. 1-3 (MD dissertation). Cambridge University, 1969.
5. Adams, F. (1849) The genuine works of Hippocrates. London: the Sydenham Society, Vol. II, p.620.
6. Browne, D. (1936) Congenital deformities of mechanical origin. Proc. Roy. Soc. Med., 29, 1409-1431.
7. Dunn, P.M. (1971) Congenital dislocation of the hips and congenital renal anomalies (Ab). Arch. Dis. Child., 46, 878.
8. Dunn, P.M. (1971) Congenital deformation following premature rupture of the membranes (Ab). Teratology, 4, 487.
9. Dunn, P.M. (1972) Congenital postural deformities: perinatal associations. Proc. Roy. Soc. Med., 65, 735-738.
10. Dunn, P.M. (1973) Congenital postural scoliosis (Ab). Arch. Dis. Child., 48, 654.
11. Dunn, P.M. (1974) Congenital postural deformities: further perinatal associations. Proc. Roy. Soc. Med., 67, 1174-1178.
12. Dunn, P.M. (1974) Congenital sternomastoid torticollis: an intrauterine postural deformity (Ab). Arch. Dis. Child., 49, 824.
13. Dunn, P.M. (1975) Growth retardation of infants with congenital postural deformities. Acta. Med. Auxol., 7, 63-68.
14. Dunn,P.M. (1976) Perinatal observations on the aetiology of congenital dislocation of the hip. Clin. Orthop., 119, 11-22.
15. Dunn, P.M. (1976) Breech presentation: maternal and fetal aetiological

factors. In: Perinatal Medicine, 5th European Congress of Perinatal Medicine. Ed. G. Rooth and L.E. Brattby. Stockholm: Almqvist and Wiksell International, pp.57-60.
16. Dunn, P.M. Congenital postural deformities. Brit. Med. Bull. 1976; 32, 71-76.
17. McKeown, T. Malformations: Introduction. In: Human malformations. Brit. Med. Bull. 1976; 32, 1-3.
18. Smith, D.W. Classification, nomenclature, and naming of morphological defects. J. Pediat. 1975; 87, 162-164.
19. Smith, D.W. Recognisable Patterns of Human Malformation. Philadelophia, W.B. Saunders Co., 1970.
20. International Statistical Classification of Diseases, Injuries and Causes of Death, 8th revision, 1965. Vol. 1, Chap. XIV, Congenital anomalies, pp. 271-290. World Health Organisation, Genève, 1967.
21. International Statistical Classification of Diseases, Injuries and Causes of Death, 9th revision, 1975. Vol. 1, Chap. XIV, Congential anomalies, pp. 417-437. World Health Organisation, Genève, 1977.
22. International Statistical Classification of Diseases and Related Health Problems, 19th revision. Vol. 1, Chap. XVII, Congenital malformations, deformations and chromosomal abnormalities, pp. 795-851. World Health Organisation, Genève,1992.
23. Smith, D.W. Recognisable Patterns of Human Deformation. Philadelphia, W.B. Saunders Co., 1981

Lessons from Royal Operations

Walford Gillison. FRCS etc.
Emeritus Consultant Surgeon
Kidderminster and City Hospital Birmingham.
Presented September 2014

INTRODUCTION

Until adequate analgesia and anaesthesia were available, surgery was limited to more superficial problems such as the drainage of abscesses, reductions of hernias or removal of superficial swellings. Alcohol and laudanum had fortunately been available for centuries. Frequently the pain of surgery had to be endured unless or until the patient fainted. Napoleon's favourite surgeon Larrey noted frozen limbs could be amputated painlessly.

Operations on anyone, let alone royalty, required the hopes that:

- Pain could be abolished,
- Infection could be avoided and
- Fluid replacement whether blood or other fluid substances were in place for the patient's survival and enable curative treatment.

RELIEF OF PAIN

Local anaesthesia

The ophthalmologist Köller demonstrated the effectiveness of cocaine on the cornea in 1884. Halstead demonstrated successful nerve blocks on the jaw in the same year. Since those early days local anaesthetic preparations have been useful to augment general anaesthesia, whether given topically by injection into the tissues, around the nerves, into the extradural space or into the spinal fluid.

General Anaesthesia

Milestones in inhalation therapy included:
1. 1840. Humphrey Davey[1] reported analgesic qualities in Nitrous Oxide but ignored by the medical profession.
2. 1842. Crawford Long removed a neck tumour using ether but did not publish until 1849.
3. 1844. Dentist Horace Wells noticed a young man under the influence of Nitrous Oxide who felt no pain after a severe blow to his shin.
4. 1846 October 16th. The first public demonstration of inhalation anaesthesia under ether by William Morton at

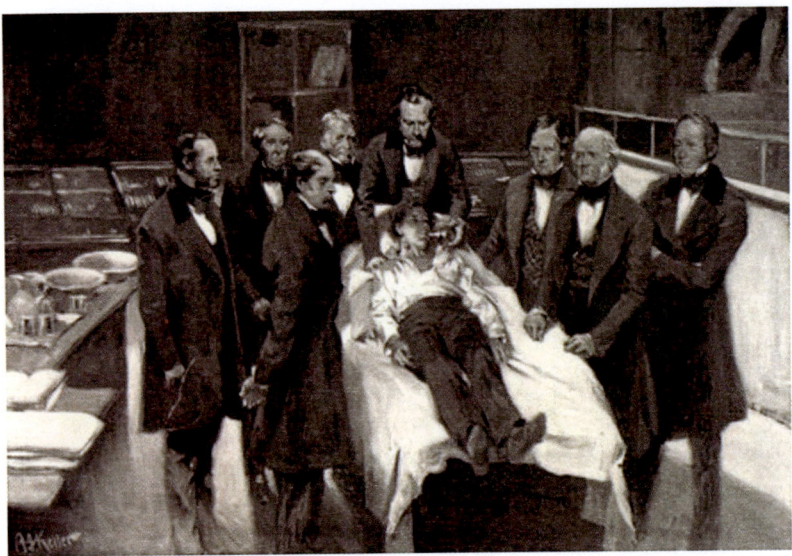

Figure 1. The re-enactment of the first public demonstration of General Anaesthesia (October 16th 1864.)
(Surgeon John Warren second right, William Morton holding the mask and the highly respected Henry Bigelow observing from far left).

the Massachusetts General Hospital[2] took place. The huge significance of this event made the original players assemble and pretend to re-enact the same operation a year later (Figure 1).
5. 1846 December 21st. Robert Liston at University College Hospital in London performed a limb amputation using ether[3].
6. 1847. Fluorens showed chloroform also had similar properties to ether[4].

As a result major advances became possible for treatment within the chest, the abdominal cavity and even inside the cranium.

BATTLES AGAINST INFECTION.

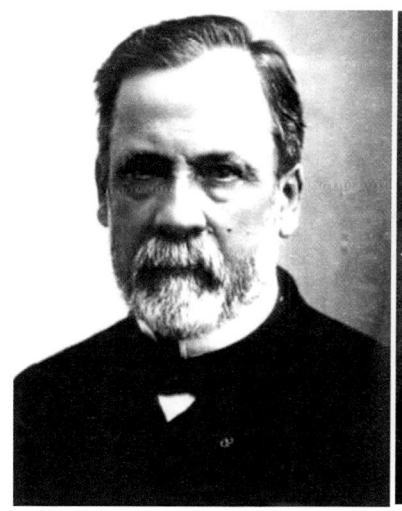
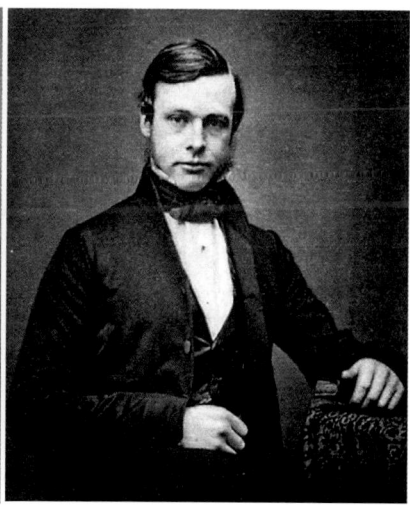

Figure 2
Louis Pasteur (1822 – 1895.)

Figure 3
Joseph Lister. 1827-1912

Pioneers had not only to wage war against infection but also against public and medical prejudice for a long time.
While Leeuwenhoek visualised protozoa and bacteria in 1693[5],

multiplication of infectious organisms was not appreciated for a long time. Spencer quoted Pasteur (Figure 2) in 1859 who showed bacteria multiplied with ease from air contamination[6], Lemaire in Paris reported the antiseptic effect of phenol on contaminated wounds[7] in1865, but Lister[8] in 1867 (Figure 3) realised and proved that the use of phenol on clean wounds reduced the risk of often fatal infection in compound fractures. (This is relevant to Henry Thompson later in the paper).

BLOOD TRANSFUSION

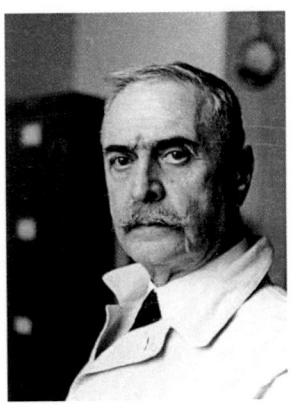

Figure 4.
Karl Lansteiner. (1866 – 1943)

Human to human blood transfusion was first performed by Blundell[9] in 1818 on two patients where one survived. Aveling in 1864 and Halstead in 1880 successfully transfused some cases before blood groups were understood.

ABO agglutinins were discovered in 1901 by Landsteiner[10] (Figure 4) which made transfusion safer. This was made even more so when he and Weiner[11] discovered the Rhesus factor in 1941. This not only made transfusion safe but enhanced survival from emergency and major operations.

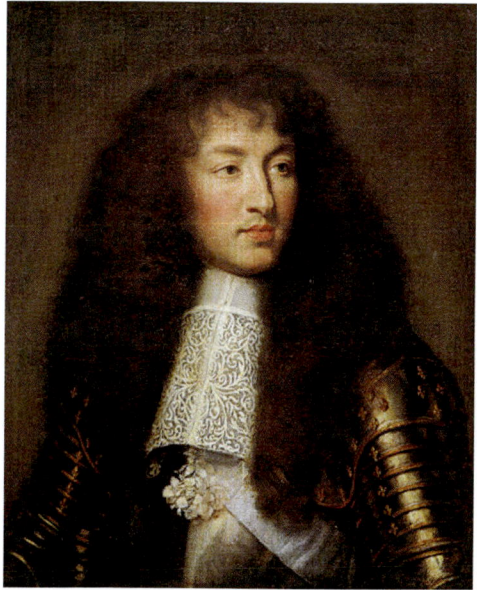

Figure 5 LOUIS XIV. (1638-1715).

ROYAL OPERATIONS

This account of Royal operations begins with the painful operation on a very distinguished King of France called "The Sun King".

Louis XIV – The "Sun King"

It was alleged that he bathed twice in his lifetime[12]; perhaps because the all-powerful Roman Church decreed that public bathing lead to promiscuity, sex and disease! His body odour was obviously well known because he perfumed his wigs and scented his clothes with sachets of herbs. A Russian ambassador said "He stunk like an animal!" Consequently audiences with the king were more popular if conducted near an open window.

The king succumbed to a peri-anal abscess in 1685 which

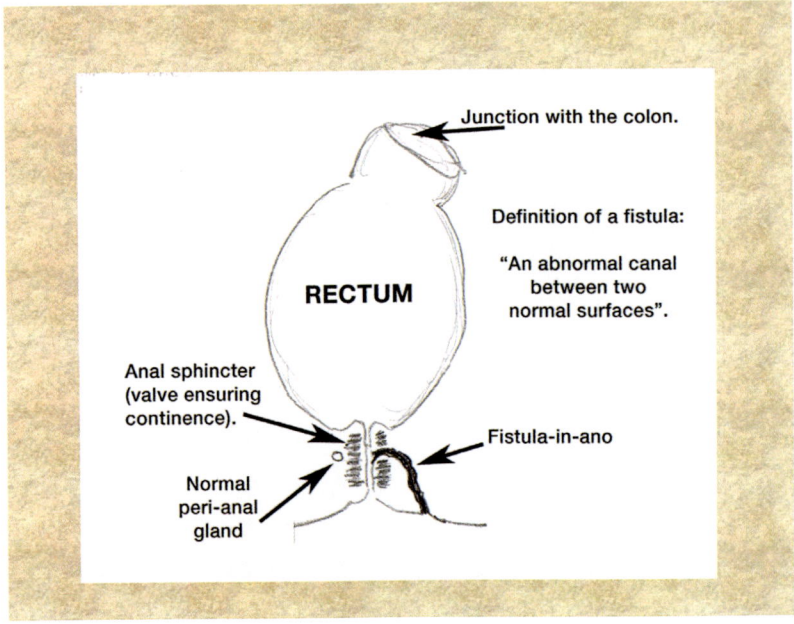

Figure 6. Fistula-in-ano

developed into a fistula (figure 6). Surgeon Charles-François Felix was summoned to Versailles to examine the king. He delayed operating for 6 months to perfect his instruments and practice his technique on a number of criminals. The operation took place on November 18th 1686 followed by four minor procedures, but the final result was excellent. The king was surprisingly a model patient.

Felix was well rewarded; he was created Baron Felix de Tassy and never touched a scalpel again!

GEORGE IV. (1762-1830).

In 1820 George IV developed a sebaceous cyst of the scalp and requested the distinguished Astley Cooper to remove it. Cooper was nervous because he had previously operated on another royal who developed erysipelas and died. Fortunately on this occasion there was no post-operative infection and Cooper received a knighthood[13.]

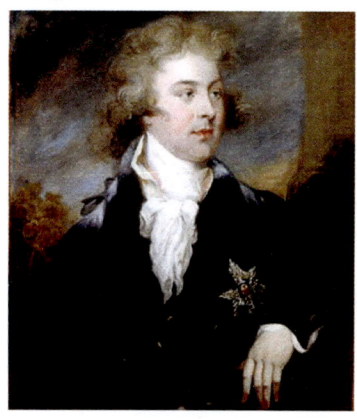

Figure 7
George IV

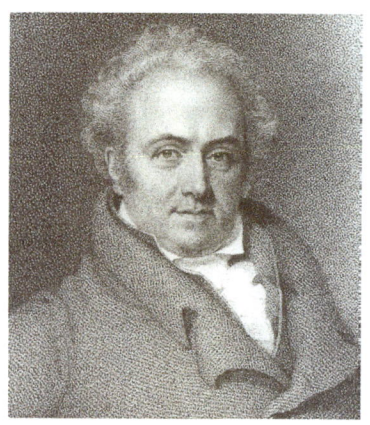

Figure 8
Astley Cooper.

LEOPOLD I. (1790-1865).

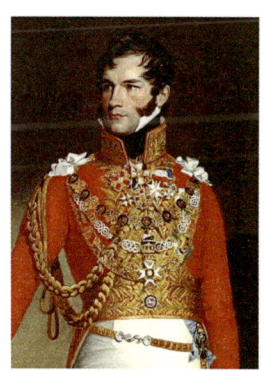

Figure 9.
Leopold I as a young man.
(1820-1904.)

Leopold, Prince of Saxe-Coburg-Gotha (figure 9) was the much loved maternal uncle of Queen Victoria and first King of the Belgians from 1831-1865. For his diplomatic skills he was regarded as the "Nestor" of Europe.

Leopold suffered from bladder stones from 1862 and was first treated by the "Father of Urology" in Europe Jean Civiale from France. Leopold endured several passages of bougies and successful lithotripsies, but each time they were complicated by severe distressing rigors for several days. In 1863 he developed recurrent symptoms on a visit to England. He was attended to by Civiale's disciple Henry Thompson (figure 10). Thompson decided to use brand new instruments on the king. This time the stones were crushed and evacuated without the usual rigors afterwards. Thompson then realised he had on this occasion used new uncontaminated equipment thus proving Lister's philosophy was correct[14].

Thompson became the first President of the British Urological Association and first president of the Cremation Society.

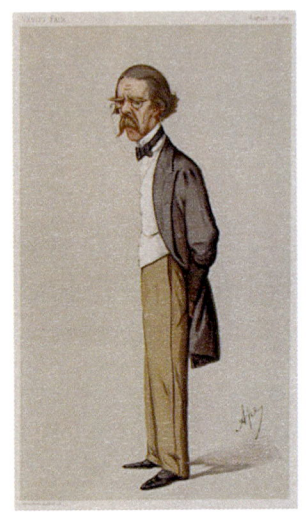

Figure 10. Henry Thompson (1790-1865).

NAPOLEON III. (1808-1871)

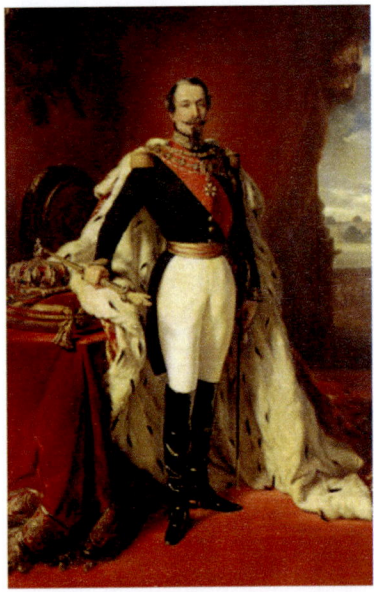

Figure 11. Napoleon III. 1808-1871

This man had a chequered career until he became the President of the Republic of France. (His cousin Napoleon II was emperor for only a few days as he died of tuberculosis.) It is known this third Napoleon had bladder symptoms for many years which he neglected and some historians wondered if his health affected his judgement during the Franco -Prussian War.

At the end of the Franco-Prussian War he was captured by Bismarck after the disastrous battle of Sedan in 1870. He was promptly exiled to Britain by the French government and soon after he suffered further attacks of urinary infection associated with renal and bladder stones. Not even Henry Thompson's skill could save him at this advanced stage[15]. Autopsy showed his bladder, ureters and renal pelves full of purulent urine.

FREDERICK III of PRUSSIA and GERMANY.

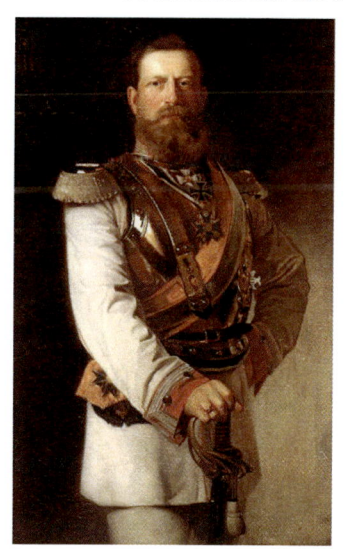
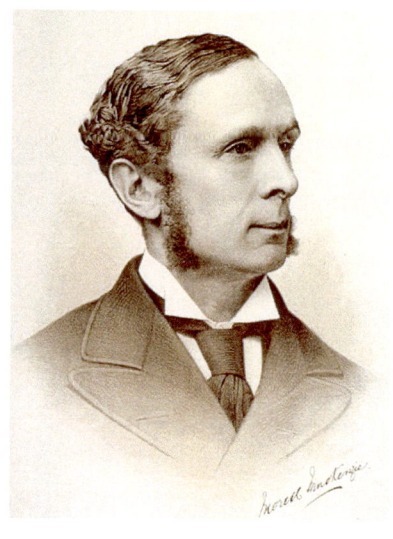

Figure 12
Frederick III. 1831-1888.

Figure 13.
Morell McKenzie.1853-1925

Frederick III was otherwise known as "Frederick the Noble" for his opposition to the attempts at dictatorship by Bismarck, but he was said to be a martinet to his own son the future Kaiser William II.

Frederick was the son of Willem I and married the British Princess Victoria. He had a brilliant military career in the Franco-Prussian War but in politics he was said to be a liberal.

He developed a hoarse voice in 1887, three biopsies by the famous Virchow failed to show cancer yet his health deteriorated. The well known British laryngologist Morell McKenzie was consulted having been recommended by Queen Victoria, but he was unable to do more than a palliative tracheostomy for the later proven cancer. Frederick's status as Kaiser lasted for only 99 days[16].

EDWARD VII. (1841-1910)
Alias "Edward the Peacemaker".

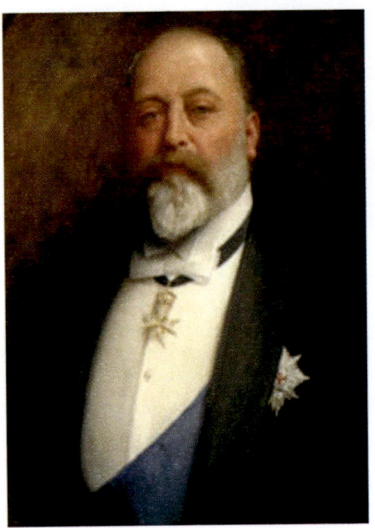
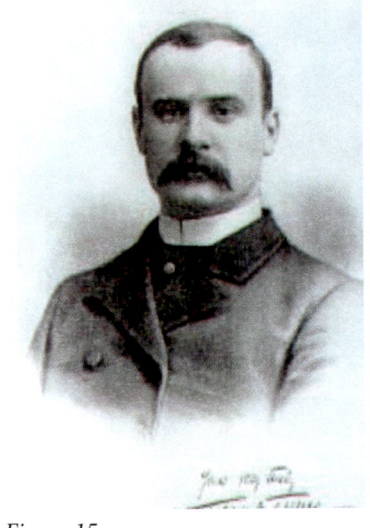

Figure 14
Edward VII 1841-1910.

Figure 15.
Frederick Treves. 1853-1923.

Edward's coronation was planned for June 26th 1902 but the ceremony had to be postponed because of abdominal pain.

He saw two different physicians on June 12th and 13th but he seemed to be getting better. London Hospital's Frederick Treves saw him on the 18th while progress continued. Following an eight course meal at Windsor on the 23rd Edward developed serious pain. Treves reviewed him and advised surgery which the king started to decline saying he promised the nation he would go to Westminster Abbey on the 26th.

Treves replied that the king would indeed go to the Abbey, not by Royal coach, but in a coffin if he did not have the operation. Reluctantly, from the king's point of view, the operation took place on June 24th. The appendiceal abscess was so bad that the appendix could not be found due to the devastating inflammation. Wisely Treves drained the presumed site of the appendix with two large rubber drains[17] and the king made a good recovery. The coronation took place on August 8th, the postponement cost the Treasury and the tax payer many thousands of pounds.

GEORGE V. (1865-1936).

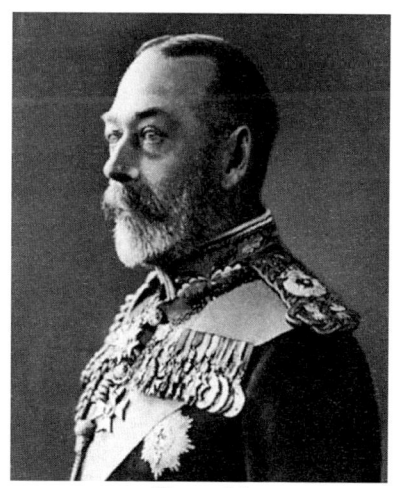
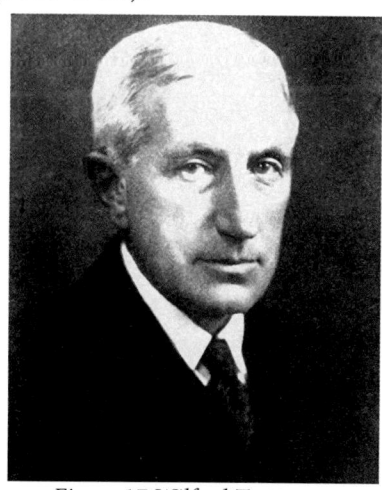

Figure 16
George V (1865-1936).

Figure 17 Wilfred Trotter
(1872-1939).

This man was a keen sailor, stamp collector, heavy smoker and because of rumours of plans for a British republic he discouraged his cousin Nicholas Alexander of Russia to receive sanctuary in Britain.

In 1928 Wilfred Trotter was called to Buckingham Palace as King George V was extremely ill. He was surgeon to University College and confirmed the diagnosis of "Empyaema Necessitans" which he treated by standard rib resection with an excellent result[18]. The king's convalescence in the seaside resort of Bognor was so successful that the town's name was changed to Bognor Regis! At first Trotter declined a knighthood; he chose to ask the king to visit his patients in the "Incurables ward". When the king agreed the ward's name was changed to "King George V ward".

Near to retirement Trotter concentrated on developing the Academic Department of Surgery instead of pursuing Private Practice. He also became President of the Royal College of Surgeons in England and of the Association of Surgeons.

GEORGE VI. 1895-1952.

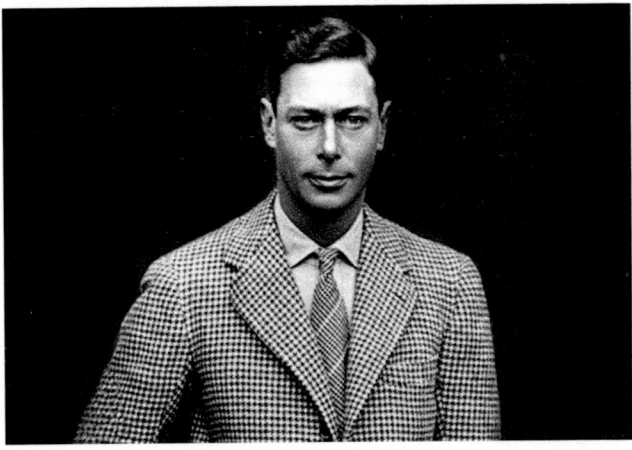

Figure 18. George VI. (1895-1952)

This reluctant king, much loved by family and country, was a

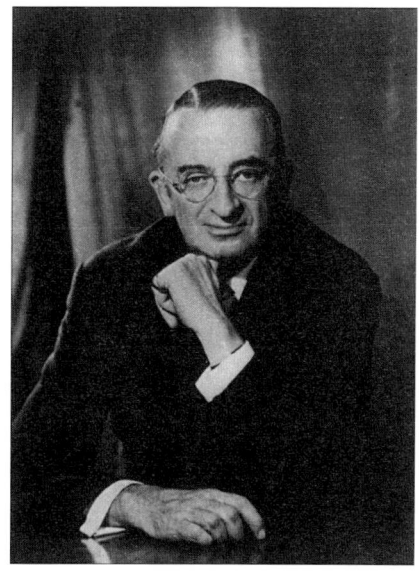
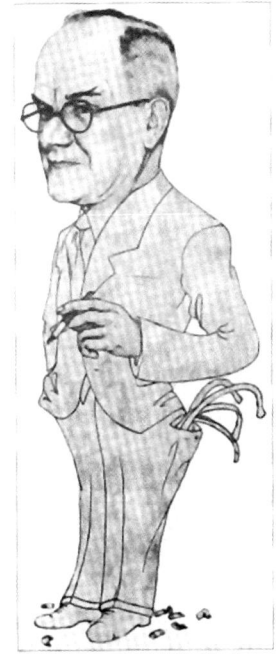

Figure 19
Horace Evans. (1903-1963).

Figure 20.
Clement Price Thomas. (1893-1973).

heavy smoker partly because of his well known nervousness and also his tendency to stammer. There was little evidence known of the complications of smoking tobacco in those days. The story of his conquering his stammer is well documented and made into a famous film in recent years.

It was no surprise that he had problems such as vascular disease of his heart and remaining arterial tree, but also he suffered recurrent chest infections. His diagnosis of pulmonary carcinoma was eventually diagnosed with the help of Horace Evans (figure 19), physician to Queen Mary and the London Hospital who happened to be visiting the Queen. Horace Evans was asked to give an opinion on the king's chest X-Ray. The resident physicians, previously unwilling to believe the king should be victim of cancer were forced to realise the situation was very grave for His Majesty and the nation.

Clement Price Thomas from the Westminster Hospital agreed to operate on the king. At first he demanded to do the operation at his own Hospital but the royal officials insisted it had to be done in the Palace. As a concession exact replicas of theatre equipment cupboards and contents from the hospital were reproduced to perfection in the palace.

On September 23rd 1951 his resident (assistant) opened the King's chest and as the tumour appeared to be operable the lung was removed. Palace officials were horrified that Mr Thomas did not open and close the chest himself. Price Thomas said he believed his procedure was the best for all his patients and could not be bettered even for his majesty. Any change in his procedure he thought would be worse for the patient. His assistants looked after the king in the palace for several days after the operation. Clement Price Thomas was knighted for his services to the King. The King did recover from the operation but not from his illnesses; he died mercifully from a heart attack in his sleep at Sandringham a few months later in February 1952[19]. It is no surprise that Sir Clement Price Thomas died of the same cancer in 1973, judging by the number of cigarette butts on the floor around him in the illustration (figure 20).

EPILOGUE.

The advent of anaesthesia converted the operating environment from First Aid stations to modern operating theatres. Surgeons have had to relinquish their statuses of "Prima Donnas" to become members of teams with other disciplines to achieve high standards of resuscitation or curative surgery whether on the battlefield or in modern medical centres.

The battle against infection significantly reduced the outcome from Lister's compound fractures from the severe risk of death or amputation. This form of surgery is now known either as "aseptic" or "anti-septic" surgery. Today increased bacterial antibiotic resistance is forcing the profession back to the drawing board. Tighter staff and patient hygiene is needed to reduce antibiotic use and new ways of fighting micro-organisms are required, such as vaccination against malaria.

Likewise blood transfusion needs to be safer still. The tragic death of tennis champion Arthur Ashe from HIV infection after blood transfusion during his cardiac operation has not been forgotten. It is hoped synthetic blood may one day be available in the future.

Charles-Francois Felix did well to cure Louis XIV. It is regrettable that the medical profession had to wait for modern proctologists to provide the exact science of dealing with fistula-in-ano. Monarchs George IV and Leopold of Belgium were fortunate and should at least be commended for their courage. Napoleon III suffered his urological problems far too long before seeking a cure for his bladder stones. Frederick III of Prussia and George VI were victims of medical attendants who did not realise that royal patients are just as vulnerable to serious disease like anyone else. Edward VII was fortunate to have a medical attendant like Treves to tell him the truth and take appropriate steps for his recovery.

REFERENCES.

1. Davy H. Researches chemical and philosophical; Chiefly concerning Nitrous Oxide. Johnson London Facsimile. London Butterworths. 1972.
2. Rudkow IM. Surgery. An Illustrated History. St. Louis. USA. Mosby 1993. p 335.
3. Zuck D. Dr Nooth and his apparatus. The role of Carbon dioxide in the 18th century. Brit. J. Anaesth. 1976. 50. 393-405.
4. Fluorens. PJ. Hebd CR. Seances. Acad Sci Paris. 1847. 24. pp 161, 253, & 340.
5. Morton LT. A Medical Biography. (Noting Antonj Leeuwenhoek's contributions 1693-1718). London: Deutch 1970: item 67.

6. Pasteur, Louis (1858). "Nouveaux faits concernant l'histoire de la fermentation alcoolique". Annales de Chimie et de Physique, 3rd Series 52: 404–418.
7. Lemaire F.J. Du Coaltar saponiné Désinfectante énergetique. Paris. Germer-Balliere, 1865.
8. Lister J. On the antiseptic principle in the practice of surgery. Brit. Med. J. 1867. Volume 2 p 246.
9. Blundell J. Observations on the transfusion of blood with a description of his Gravitator. Lancet 1928. 2 321-4.
10. Landsteiner K. 1901. Haematology landmark papers of the twentieth century. Lichtman et al. London Academic Press 2000.
11. Landsteiner K & Weiner AS. An agglutinable factor in human blood recognised by immune sera from human blood. Proceedings of the Society of Experimental Biology and Medicine. 1940. 43. 223-4.
12. Perez S. The hygiene of Louis XIV. www.ncbi.nlm.nih.gov./pubmed/18549079.
13. Wikipedia https://en.wikipedia.org/wiki/Astley_Cooper.
14. Ellis H. Famous Operations. Harwal Publishing Company Ltd. Media. Pennsylania. Ch 13. p 102.
15. Ellis H. Famous Operations. Harwal Publishing Company Ltd. Media. Pennsylvania. Ch 13. p 106.
16. Morell McKenzie. Case of Emperor Frederick III. Classic Reprint Series. Forgotten Books. June 20th 2012.
17. Michael KH Crumplin. Pioneers in Surgical Gastroenterology. Edited Walford Gillison and Henry Buchwald. Tfm Publishing Ltd. Shrewsbury SY5 6LX 2007. Ch 12. p 209.
18. Ellis H. Famous Operations. Harwal Publishing Company Ltd. Media. Pennsylvania. Ch 15. p 122.
19. Obituary. King George VI. Brit Med J. 1952. 1. 386.

A short history of old age pensions
Growing old (dis)gracefully

BRUNO BUBNA-KASTELIZ
President 2012-2016
Presented September 2015

Here are some quotes about old age which are relevant to the talk I am about to give and which suggest that retirement was not in the past, and may not be in the future, necessarily all that it's cracked up to be.

Cast me not off in the time of my old age
When I am old and greyheaded,
O God, forsake me not.
Psalm 71

"Had I served God as diligently as I have served the King,
He would not have given me over in my grey hairs"
Cardinal Wolsey

"Do not go gentle into that good night,
Old age should burn and rave at close of day;
Rage, rage against the dying of the light."
Dylan Thomas

We all have a sense of uncertainty about the future and try to guard against any unwelcome surprises by making arrangements to insure ourselves in some way, so that when old age or infirmity hits us we are prepared, if not spiritually or emotionally, at least financially. Even in ancient civilisations we can see the beginnings of such insurance, with the grant of pensions in ancient Greece for instance. An old age pensioner who lived in the Palestine area in 562 B.C. features in the Bible, although we don't know his name. As for England, it was recorded that Henry III awarded one of his army sergeants an old age pension in 1269. And so-called 'perpetual hereditary pensions' were a feature of mediaeval and later times and were commonly held by the favourites of the Crown. These were really un-earned salaries for sinecures – e.g. in Charles II's time the Duke of Grafton (one of his illegitimate sons) was given the title of Keeper of Mines for what was then a very large annual pension of £4000. I was acquainted with the grandson of Ferdinand de Lesseps, the builder of the Suez Canal, and his off-spring had been receiving a life-time pension from the French government until the 1960s.

The idea of monetary support for those too old or sick to work really started in Britain in the 8th century with the 'Guilds' under King Alfred. These "...bound Guild Bretheren to mutual assistance for the aid of the poor, helpless, sick stranger, pilgrims, prisoners and burial of the dead". The Guilds were organisations or alliances in certain localities, not related to mercantile or professional pursuits, but recognised by King Alfred and his successor King Athelstan. There is a history of soldiers and sailors receiving sums on discharge from service even as far back as the Middle Ages. Later there was the so-called 'Chatham Chest' which was a pension scheme set up in 1590 for disabled seamen and was financed by members' contributions which were deducted from their pay. Many of the rich in the Middle Ages could book themselves a room and board in a monastery when they got old and pay the monks to say masses for their souls after death. Civil servants and public officials needed to be kept sweet by the King so they would do his business, but we know that many of them used their power to squeeze favours and bribes out of people and this was reckoned to be part of the 'perks' of the job, although in fact constituted a private pension scheme. Most artisans and certainly artists who needed patronage to survive could, if they pleased their patrons, receive personal pensions, viz. Titian from the Doge of Venice or Michaelangelo from the Pope &c. In the 16th century, Henry VIII assumed that the aged would receive voluntary alms. This assumption was based on the fact that the monasteries had provided social relief and material support to the sick, aged and incapacitated 'in the community' throughout mediaeval England. The wealth accumulated over many centuries by the religious houses was due in part to the insistence of the clergy that the well-off paid for having absolution from their confessors and penitential masses said, or making donations to the monasteries or convents in their wills [rather like solicitors suggesting charitable will-making nowadays!]. The confiscation by Henry VIII of monastic wealth in the Dissolution resulted in the loss of this pre-existing social support and there was an inevitable re-distribution of this wealth to the middle class and Court favourites. Attempts to deal with the idle, the incapacitated or the aged, and now destitute people, became a feature of the landscape throughout the 16th and 17th century and led to the Statute of Poor Law in 1601 in the last year of Elizabeth I's reign. Every parish was to appoint an overseer whose duty it was to levy rates for the relief of the poor and aged. The rates were also to be spent on apprenticeships of children whose parents could not maintain them, as well as providing work for the able-bodied and assisting those who could not work due to infirmity or old age. Relief was divided into in- and out-relief, meaning that a person who needed institutional care would receive in-relief in a workhouse or alms house and that a person who merely required financial assistance got out-relief. It is interesting that this principle hardly changed in the next 300 years of the Poor Law's administration.

The monarchs who followed Elizabeth made alms-giving increasingly compulsory. By the time of Charles I, he and his bishops managed in spite of the resistance from, rather than with the help of, Parliament to get pensions for the aged poor. In 1630 the first change to the 1601 Poor Law occurred – providing support for not just those incapacitated by age but also younger incapacitated adults. The trouble was that there were always objectors who saw any charity given to the younger poor as taking away the will to work from those who might be naturally indolent.

This worked well for a generation or so but then the aftermath of the Civil War saw chronic unemployment on a national scale. Cromwell and the Puritans looked on the poor with stern eyes. They thought that relief for widows, orphans and the aged was a matter for charity, not Parliament. The result was the construction of more workhouses and alms houses in that period but little financial support for the elderly. After 1662, the introduction of the law of 'settlement' aggravated the situation. The receiving of assistance was based on parishes and a man was deemed to have settlement in a parish and be entitled to relief if he had lived in the same parish for 3 years or been born, married or owned property in that parish. If settlement was not proven then the applicant could be turned out and sent back to his 'own' parish.

Daniel Defoe was among other things (such as writer of the first English 'novel' and a state spy) a Pensions Officer and wrote in 1697: "All sorts of labouring people of honest repute shall pay down 6 pence on entry [into the pension scheme] and from hence 1 shilling a quarter". He set up 'tables' of predicted lifespans and thought that 100,000 subscribers would finance the scheme, so that "…no creature so miserable or so poor should claim subsistence as their due, nor ask it for charity". Fifty years later, in 1757, coal heavers working on the Thames were able "…to make provision for themselves, as shall be sick, lame or past their labour, and for widows and orphans" by virtue of an Act of Parliament setting up what became to be known as Box Clubs. Soon similar arrangements we made by boat skippers and keel-men in the coal trade on the Wear in County Durham. Presumably this was as a result of the importance of these workers in the burgeoning industries supporting the beginnings of the Industrial Revolution.

In the time of George III, the matter of pensions for 'top people' was regulated by Parliament for the remuneration of some public service holders – the so-called 'Consolidated Fund', or what later came to be known as the 'Civil List', by which of course we also pay the Royal Family. The Political Pensions Act of 1869 was introduced to deal with pensions for Ministers and certain parliamentary officers but the act went into abeyance in 1924. This Act was then revived and modified in two further Acts in 1937 and 1939, which identified the pension of the Lord Chancellor, for instance, as well as judges and highest ranking officers in the Forces. Incidentally, the 'hereditary pensions' were finally voted out in Parliament in 1887 after a report of the Select Committee on Hereditary Pensions (chaired by the famous social reformer Charles Bradlaugh).

Throughout the 18th century, several experiments in reform for giving assistance were tried - workhouses for indoor relief and farming out the poor as cheap labour for contracted farmers for outdoor relief, all supplemented from the rates. This of course put an increasing burden on rate payers and there was an in-built variability of the amounts of relief given, according to the situation in the parishes. Finally, the so-called 'Speenhamland system' became more widely spread. A rule was made in 1795 by magistrates meeting in the Pelican Inn, Speenhamland in Berkshire that allowances should be on a sliding scale regulated by the local price of bread. For the ordinary man in the 18th century who became destitute through unemployment or incapacity to work, the state supplied nothing but the workhouse or jail. The trouble was that the Box Clubs and their like became increasingly suspect to the government of the day and they were made illegal. The government was suspicious of combinations of workmen which could possibly foment disaffection and rioting. At the same time in that century the government was in a cleft stick - trying by repeated legislation to regulate the enormous quantities of gin drunk by the poorest of the population [think of Hogarth's picture entitled 'Gin Alley'] and which of course affected their health and productivity – but not wanting to reduce the enormous revenue from the tax on gin. Parliament encouraged the setting up of what were called Friendly Societies in two Parliamentary Acts in 1793 - the Gilbert Act and the Rose Act. In 1796, William Pitt as Chancellor of the Exchequer proposed an alternative of setting up parochial funds raised by voluntary contributions and supported by the rates for funding relief, because he felt that the Poor law was 'burdensome and degrading' but nothing came of his proposal.

By the early 19th century the expenditure on the administration of Poor Law relief was becoming crippling on the parishes. It has to be remembered that this was just after the expensive prolonged war with France and a substantial loss or disablement of working-age men. In 1816, the cost to the parish was 13s/3d per annum per head of population. In the meantime, craft bodies and Friendly Societies had set up funds for social support separate from the Poor Law and in 1819 the Friendly Societies Act was passed to regulate them. This provided contributions on the principle of mutual insurance for advanced age and widowhood. The State Agency Act of 1833 allowed purchase of annuities, immediate or deferred, through saving banks to a maximum of £20 and minimum of £4, via the Post Office. However the financial position of the Friendly Societies was precarious and was subject to fraud and embezzlement. From 1793 to 1876 there were 38,315 of these Societies, of which one third suffered financial collapse in the later period, largely because they used the wrong actuarial figures, because mortality rates had begun to improve, so they were forced to pay out for longer periods than expected. In the 1870s many Friendly Societies re-invented themselves and called themselves Consolidated Societies, based on better actuarial figures. Unfortunately, in the switch of names and administration, many older contributors lost all the money they had set aside [shades of Robert Maxwell or badly invested pension funds today!].

The New Poor Law of 1834 swept away unrestricted out-relief and grouped parishes together into what were called Unions. These Unions undertook a massive building programme between 1834 and about 1850 of building workhouses and infirmaries and some 200 were built in England and Wales. These New Poor Law institutions formed the stock of many cottage hospitals and geriatric and psychiatric units around the country after 1948 of course! The Unions were each under a Board of Guardians, with strong central authority to enforce a uniform policy. The cardinal principle was that relief should only be given to the able-bodied poor and their dependents in a well-regulated workhouse under conditions inferior to the humblest labourer outside. Men and women, even spouses and their children were separated in different parts of the building. These drastic measures of deterrence naturally provoked widespread popular discontent and was indeed one of the grievances which played a part in the Chartist Riots. The upside was that it did somewhat reduce the volume and cost of pauperism, at least for a time. But the deterrent principle was continued further in that 'able-bodied tests' were applied to the unemployed, particularly to 'casual' applicants. This was the name given to the roving vagrants who applied to use the 'casual wards' of the workhouse for overnighting. The 'tests' consisted of stone-breaking – for instance, the stone floors of the individual cells in the separate 'casual ward' building to the right of the road entrance at St. Martin's Hospital in Bath until the recent upgrading to residential flats, had grills set in them and a pile large stones in the corner of the cell had to be broken down by hand to go through the grill for the 'casual' to obtain his gruel and night's rest. This of course was not only cruel but uneconomical. This was cruel for the honest work-seeker but utterly useless from the point of view of reforming the work-shy. Moreover, the workhouse mostly contained able-bodied persons who were left to twiddle their thumbs in demoralising idleness. Workhouses also contained children who were usually ill-tended and poorly educated, mixed in with elderly paupers. The care provided to the inmates of the infirmaries and 'chronic sick' wards, often containing a mixture of the mentally disturbed and what were then called 'the backward, imbeciles and idiots' as well as the physically disabled, was a scandal.

Gladstone as Chancellor of the Exchequer became interested in the administration of the Poor Law funds. He wanted to make government less financially beholden to the banks and the City, which of course was then and ever since, never achieved. He set up Post Office Saving Banks, which for the first time gave the public small annuities secure from risks of fraud or bankruptcy. This scheme only finally folded in 1928. In the Royal Commission on Friendly Societies set up in 1871, the idea of a national, state-run Friendly Society to complement the Post Office Savings Banks was urged on the government. Of these two ideas, the first was not well advertised nor sufficiently taken up by the public and the second was scuppered by the Association of Friendly Societies who lobbied hard against any reform.

An attempt in 1878 by a Rev. William Blackley to set up a system of National Insurance run by the Post Office was also bitterly attacked by the Friendly Societies. Another advanced idea put forward by his associate reformer Charles Hookham to consider non-contributors benefiting from a pension in old age, irrespective of savings - in short a right for all, not to be considered like the dole – was thrown out, despite public support. A word about the Reverend Blackley: he was an interesting man who had been tutored in his teens in Brussels by a Polish refugee and then attended Dublin University. His Irish eloquence, warmth and witty humour made him popular with leading politicians but unpopular with the Friendly Societies. He was fluent in several languages and through his widespread contacts was aware of legislation taking shape on the Continent. His views, which he expounded freely, had a direct effect on the promotion of old age pension schemes in Denmark, New Zealand and Australia. Bismarck, the 'Iron Chancellor' of Germany, regarded social unrest as an evil and the insecurity and anxiety of the working man when he contemplates an impoverished old age as one of the main causes of unrest. As he put it: *"Remove that anxiety and you remove their hatred and avert more serious troubles...* [I suspect he was influenced by the 1848 European Revolution] and later, he said: *"Why should regular soldiers and officials have pensions but not the soldier of labour?"* Bismarck managed to get an Invalidity and Old Age Insurance Act through the Reichstag in 1889, which asked for equal contributions from both employer and employee to help fund it. He had also realised that the government would initially have to subsidise the fund to pay off those who were entitled at the age of 70 but had not contributed for long.

Blackley felt that dependence on the Poor Law to supply the wants of the aged poor in England was both unjust and degrading – unjust, in that it was inequitable and unfair to ratepayers and thrifty working men, who were supporting the shiftless and thriftless; degrading, as it demeaned and labelled a man and his family as inadequate or worse. [The pamphlets on his ideas which he had published are available to read in the Reference section of Bath Library!] Naturally the Government did the usual thing when faced with a problem it wanted to go away, it set up a Royal Commission in 1891 which was startled to discover that while only 8% of people under 60 years were receiving relief, 25% of both men and women over 60 were in receipt of poor relief, so the cause was clearly not intemperate living but the poverty and infirmity of old age. Further Commissions were organised to "consider whether any alterations in the Poor law were desirable..." A final report in 1895 considered three alternative schemes for funding old age pensions, namely Imperial taxation, compulsory insurance and state-aided insurance. However the government took no action and yet another Royal Commission of 1899 proposed several sensible alternatives after only 3 months' deliberation but the Boer War intervened and again nothing happened. After the war George Barnes, an early trade unionist activist managed to get Lloyd George on his side. The latter famously said he wanted to "lift the shadow of the workhouse from the homes of the poor" but no material progress was made.

Then in 1908 Prime Minister Campell-Bannerman introduced an Old Age Pensions Bill which provided between one shilling and 5 shillings a week to men over 70, as long as they weren't earning more than 12 shillings a week or £31.10s a year. There were constraints as to who was eligible: only those of British nationality or UK domicile for over 20 years. Those who were already in receipt of Poor Law relief, prisoners whose crime could not be offset by a fine, those convicted under the Inebriate Act 1898 or who were defined under the Lunacy Act 1851 and lastly those who were shown to be consistently work-shy, did not qualify. In addition, the spouse's income was counted towards the couple's joint income ceiling, so they received less if their joint income came to more than £31.10s. This Bill did not however get on the Statute books. Another Royal Commission in 1909 (by now no. 5) demanded drastic reform of the Poor Law in a new Bill. There was, however, criticism of this Bill in that, although the local authorities could take over the functions of the Board of Guardians it would not finally abolish the Poor Law either in name or function and duplication and overlapping of administration would result in chaos. The government was therefore not disposed to support the Bill. Finally in 1911, Lloyd George brought about the introduction of the Old Age Pensions Bill, but which unfortunately still had quite a few of the prior disqualifications in it. One has to remember that this means-tested pension was for 70-year-old men only when the average life expectancy was only forty-eight! Attempts at bringing in any additional reforms were abandoned because of the onset of World War 1.

However, WW1 did change peoples' attitude to many things, including working women, workers' rights and responsibilities. These social changes were coupled with an overall reduction in the number of working men at the War's end. A Ministry of Pensions was formed in 1916, which ordered a re-examination of relief and pensions under Sir Donald Maclean (father of the spy of Burgess & Maclean notoriety). This proposal would result in the transfer of Poor Law administration, maternal and childrens' services as well as mental health to the Local Authority, Public Health and Local Education Service, but these reforms were implemented only slowly and piecemeal over the following years. Then came the huge numbers of unemployed and General Strike of 1926 and the demand on relief overwhelmed the Boards of Guardians who were still partially responsible for the administration of relief. Outdoor relief was a dead letter since Board members ignored restrictions imposed by the Local Authorities, who were officially surcharged and the Ministers turned a blind eye. In fact it was clear that it wasn't socialism or fascism which dictated the opposing views in this political spat but the folly of putting new wine into old bottles.

The year 1919 saw the first link made between pension contributions and national insurance. However the cut-off age was still 70 for both sexes and means testing was only modified in 1924 by a contributory insurance system. The number of people receiving old age pensions in 1922 was 705,678 but had climbed to over one million by 1926.

Finally in 1929, Neville Chamberlain, as Minister of Health managed to get the Local Authority Act passed which abolished the Board of Guardians, transferred their powers to the Public Assistance Committees of the Local Authorities under the control of the Ministry of Health. This formed the last of the Poor Law Acts of 1930. The pensionable age had been reduced to 65 for both sexes in 1925 (womens' pensionable age did not reduce to 60 until 1940).

Pension books were issued for the first time but those elderly living in Poor Law institutions had their pensions collected by an 'agent' because if they received their relief in the institution the Local Authority took it over 'to defray costs of care' and these persons were allowed two shillings a week as a 'personal allowance' [remember that at present pensioners admitted to hospital have to inform the Social Services and some benefits such as Attendance Allowance and Carers' allowance are stopped]. Some improvements and a few restrictions in pensions occurred under various post-World War II administrations but much more recent reform has been grudging, retrograde or punitive, partially due to the cumulative negative effects of increased longevity, low birth rates and fiscal parsimony we are seeing latterly.

I leave you with two contrasting decennial population bar charts and the prediction that state old age pensions will be unlikely to be available for our great-grandchildren, or perhaps even our grandchildren, as the ratio of retired to working population reaches 1:<1.

Population profile per decade - men & women - 1900

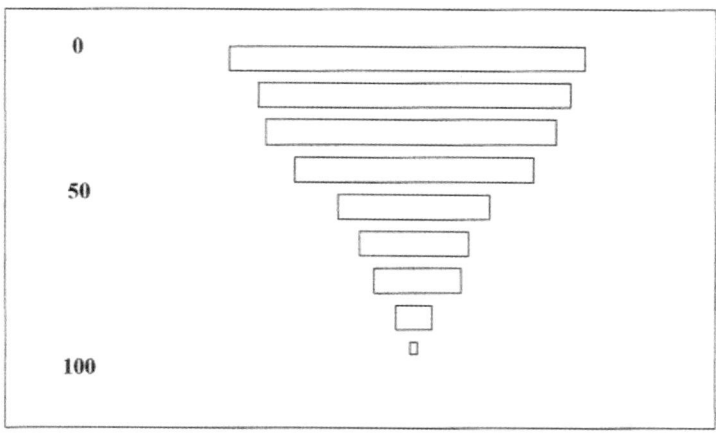

Population profile per decade - men & women - 2000

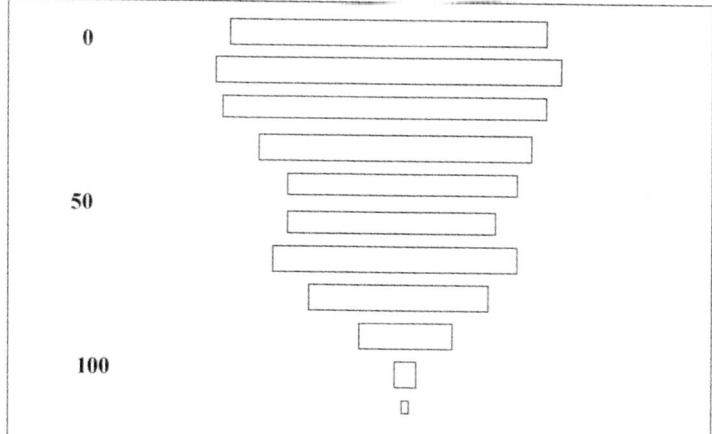

A History of Inebriacy in Bristol

PETER CARPENTER
Presented September 2015

I've talked on inebriacy in Bristol before when talking about the work of the Burdens and Brentry Hospital. Today I want to take a more long-term view of the different institutions and services in Bristol. I've only found a few and would welcome help from others in identifying more.

I'm very aware that Dr Crabbe is in the audience today who wrote a thesis on women and alcohol at the turn of last century. I hope that she can give a talk at a future time.

Dr Bubna-Kasteliz earlier referred to drunkenness being seen as a social problem. Hogarth's 'Gin Lane' reinforces this image and attitude. However the Nineteenth Century saw a move for it to be seen as a medical disorder. In 1804 Thomas Trotter, a Scottish physician recently retired from the fleet, published his 'Essay on Drunkenness' which declared that *"the habit of Drunkenness is a disease of the mind."* Twenty five years later, in 1829 the Temperance movement started in Glasgow.

A major campaigner for change was Donald Dalrymple. Originally a Norwich surgeon and the proprietor of a lunatic asylum, he considered alcohol a potent cause of insanity, which was a common view as evidenced by many of the tables of causation published by medical officers. In 1869 he went to the States and looked at their Inebriate asylums, in particular one that claimed a cure rate of 40%. Next year he became the MP for Bath and was in a strong position to advocate for treatment of habitual drunkards.

His first big debate on this subject in 1870 did not go well with the Home Secretary reluctant to legislate on this matter, saying:

"He [Mr Bruce] could understand that an institution such as that at Boston, where people voluntarily engaged to submit to a certain discipline for a certain time, might be productive of advantage; but he thought it impossible to call upon Parliament to pass a law by which person affected with drunkenness should be kept in a sort of gaol till, in the opinion of physicians who had charge of them, they were sufficiently masters of themselves to be liberated.

...it would not be possible ... to give a certificate that a drunkard who had been kept from stimulants was sufficiently master of himself to be trusted not to get drunk again. This was an entirely new step, and though that was not reason why it should not be considered, he believed it was one of a most dangerous kind....

It might be a great advantage to society to detain those men who lived upon follies of youth; and, in fact, there were many other pests of society and of themselves who might, no doubt, advantageously be immured and kept in confinement for ever; but, as yet, Parliament had not thought fit to pass an Act to render such a proceeding legal."

Similarly Bucknill in 1878 attacked the bill as too simplistic and pointed out two distinct types of habitual drunkards: those where it was a vice where reform was by moral methods and could not be cured by any medical treatment; alongside those where it was a form of insanity and the person needed medical care and treatment and not a moral cure.

Dalrymple's campaign resulted in the 1879 Habitual Drunkard Act which allowed a habitual drunkard to sign themselves into a licensed retreat in front of a magistrate for 13 months. They also had to pay for their time in the retreat. This mainly catered for the wealthy under family pressure to change and did in fact produce a respectable cure rate.

There were also private retreats "not under the act" which had voluntary inmates.

One suspects several of the private asylums acted as such private retreats for one or two patients. These would have been Bailbrook House in Bath, Brislington House and Northwood Asylum. The place dedicated to alcohol treatment that advertised was Dunmurry in Goodeve Road operated by Dr James Stewart who was an ex-Naval Surgeon. It was advertising by 1886 and in 1910 he advertised having relinquished his work and that he was looking for alternatives.

This home was one from gentlefolk and as part of his publications he published on the correct treatment of inebriated gentlefolk which includes the following advice.

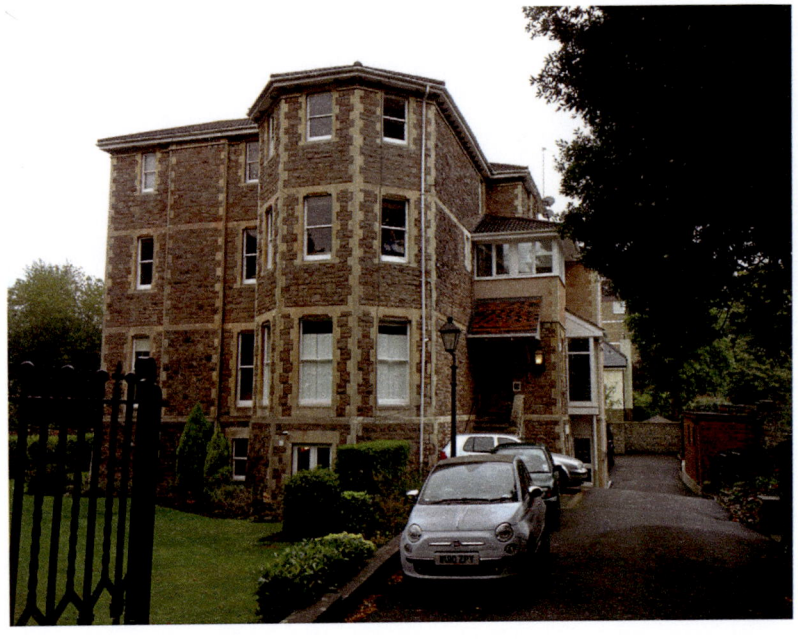

Figure 1.
Dunmurry House, Goodeve Road in 2015

"What ought to be his treatment there? If the resident physician be a man of experience he will cut off absolutely and entirely from the very first all alcoholic stimulants, whether in the shape of beer or claret or anything else.

The depression from which inebriates are generally suffering when they first reach a home requires the frequent administration of egg and milk, beef-tea, milk and lime water, soda and milk and other easily assimilated beverages, taken every hour and a half at first and gradually reduced in frequency.

The sleeplessness from which almost all inebriates suffer at first is best treated by draft composed of 20 minims of the solution of bimeconate of Morphia with 10 to 15 grains of choral, alternated for a few nights with other hypnotics. ....

As the strength of body returns gentle exercise ought to be insisted on, increased gradually till at least 8 or 10 miles a day for a gentlemen, or 5 miles for a lady, can be accomplished with ease. [If he has no hobby he should take one up.]

Here I will take the opportunity to protest against the mistaken idea, ... that by the exhibition of such drugs as capsicum you can destroy the craving for alcohol, or at least keep it under. You may perhaps smother it for a while by repeated doses of the perchloride of iron, or one of the class of drugs to which capsicum belongs, or possibly by what was for a while so much vaunted – a particular sort of bark, or the recently recommended Strychnine "cure"; but my experience [is you are] ... only substituting one enslavement for another.

The same remark applies to some extent to aerated beverages. Without absolutely interdicting them I recommend to my patients to do without them, to drink plain filtered water at their dinner and take plenty of milk with either tea or coffee. It should be drilled into the minds of drink-cravers that the addition of a little lime water will make milk digestible by even the most delicate stomach.

The regular meals in the Home for Inebriates ought to be four in number besides afternoon tea, the latter being invariably very weak. [there should not be more than six inmates (of which 2 should be women under attention of the wife)]*

THE ROYAL VICTORIA HOME

The first big licensed retreat in Bristol was set up by the Revd Burden and his first wife in 1895. This was the Royal Victoria Home situated just outside the entrance to Bristol prison and still there today used as accommodation for staff. Revd Harold Nelson Burden had come to Bristol as secretary of the Church of England Temperance Society and linked with the Prison Gate Mission. He organised the creation of the Royal Victoria Home operated by a charitable committee of local notables. It was for poor women only and had such curative pastimes as basket weaving, laundry and straw plaiting. In addition it appears to have also been offered as an alternative to prison for some women. Interestingly it backs onto a pub.

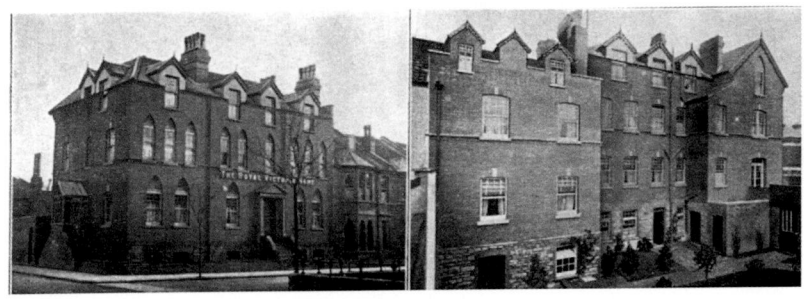

Figure 2.
The Royal Victoria Home

THE INEBRIATE ACT

In 1898 another Act was passed, now called the Inebriate Act, using the new medical term. It enabled compulsory detention of Habitual Drunkards for three years in a licensed reformatory if they are either convicted four times in a year of drunkenness or guilty of an offence punishable with imprisonment. The treatment used in reformatories though continued to be moral and not medical.

The Revd Burden spearheaded the opening of Brentry House and grounds as the Royal Victoria Homes. This was an amalgam of the original charity running the retreat and of councils who purchased beds. It also used the original Royal Victoria Home as the female admission unit. The place had a financial crisis shortly after opening and the councils had to bail it out. The Burdens left but bought the original Royal Victoria Home and went on to create the National Institutions for Inebriates, creating over 400 beds around the country.

Brentry Reformatory continued with a fairly turbulent life due to its recalcitrant inmates - there were several riots requiring police intervention and one mass escape when over 30 walked out pursued by the police. As part of this the place had its own police station - we were still using the police cells as offices in 2000 when we closed the building.

The problem with the reformatories was that they did not cure the inmates admitted against their will. In 1908 London was running out of enthusiasm for them with the magistrates complaining they were just expensive prisons and the inmates returned to drink on their release. London stopped buying beds in reformatories and as they became less popular the reformatories around the country closed over the next eight years with all the reformatories transferring their inmates to Brentry as they became unviable. Brentry ended up being the first and last reformatory in England with the last inmate leaving in 1922. Most of the empty reformatories were reused as Mental Deficiency Colonies. In 1912 there was an attempt to bring in a new act where one could commit yourself to stay sober and if you relapsed be placed in a reformatory for two years, but this bill failed to reach law.

The failure to be cured in a reformatory was put down to the Inebriate being mentally defective. The Mental Deficiency Act allowed an Inebriate to be admitted as a mental defective, but I have not come across any case so admitted.

One man I would like to mention because he shows the closeness between the Home Office and the Burdens is Robert Welsh Braithwaite. He was the first medical superintendent at Dalrymple House and advocated keeping after-care records to show success rates and supported the Inebriate Reformation and After-care Association. With the 1898 Inebriate Act he became the first Inspector of Reformatories and with the 1913 Mental Deficiency Act the first inspector of Mental Deficiency Colonies, and then a medical commissioner for the Board of Control but he clearly kept close links with the Burdens and acted as an advisor. In 1919 he was witness for the quiet wedding of Harold Burden to Rosa Gladys Williams, and when he retired from the Board of Control in 1926 he became director of medical services at Stoke Park, run by the Burdens, though he never effectively took up this role as he died three years later.

The mental health acts after this excluded drinking alcohol as a cause for detention, probably because of the failure of compulsory treatment under the Inebriates Act. Alcohol treatment appears to have comprised general practice intervention and the occasional detox and possibly psychotherapy in private hospitals.

The next treatment force was the self-help group, Alcoholics Anonymous which started in the States in 1935 and reached London in 1947. It spread quickly around England and in 1953 the first meeting in Bristol was held in the Full Moon Pub with a Bath group in 1955, and a Wells Hospital group by 1960.

THE ROBERT SMITH UNIT

In 1980 Bristol NHS created its first alcohol treatment unit, namely the Robert Smith unit which opened in the old Hospital opened by Elizabeth Dunbar, Hospital in Clifton, next to Mortimer House [now called Dunbar House]. At that time several community treatment teams were starting around the country, some using an AA model and some, such as Leicester where I worked, used a social drinking model.

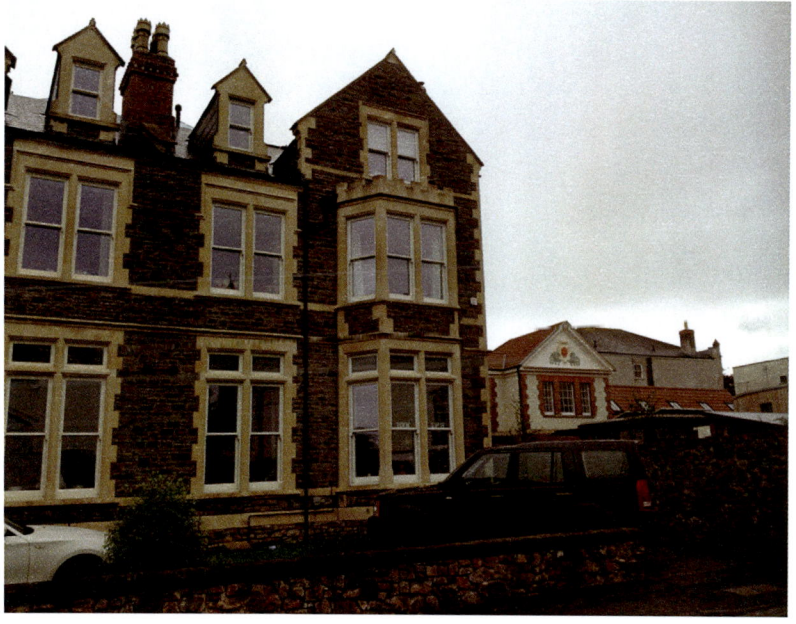

Figure 3.
The Robert Smith site at 12 Mortimer Road in 2015. Stables in the distance.

Originally The Robert Smith Unit was to be an inpatient unit but the money for beds was withdrawn just before it opened so it was forced to become a community treatment centre. It was named after Dr Bob, the founder of AA and it was the AA model that it used for treatment. Dr Tony Willam was the first consultant. In about 1995 it moved to the old Public Health premises in 12 Mortimer Road adjacent to Mortimer House and not into the stables of Mortimer House as I've always thought. In 2009 it moved again to Colston Fort as part of the Bristol Specialist Drug and Alcohol Service. At that time 20-25 people were attending Robert Smith unit every day.

CONCLUSION

So in conclusion the 19th-century saw alcohol abuse becoming a medical disease with attempts to cure it with moral treatment. Compulsory treatment of the unwilling failed miserably and this has affected mental health act legislation for the following century.

In the 20th century it stopped being seen as a priority for mental illness hospitals unless you paid them and the AA took over as a force for self treatment with a community treatment unit starting almost by default in Bristol in 1980.

In discussions after the talk members recalled that patients would be sent to two other local units outside of Bristol: Broadway Lodge, in Oldmixon near Weston-super-Mare, which opened in 1974 as a private addictions unit offering 12 Step rehabilitation [and claims to be the first in England to do so] and Clouds House in East Knoyle in Wiltshire which opened in about 1983 and also offered rehabilitation based on the 12 step programme.

REFERENCES

1. Dr James Stewart: The treatment of Inebriety in the higher and educated classes" Quarterly Journal of Inebriety Jan 1886.

The Rise and Fall of Childbed Fever
PETER M. DUNN, MA, MD, FRCP, FRCOG, FRCPCH
*Emeritus professor of Perinatal Medicine
and Child Health, University of Bristol, UK
e-mail: P.M.Dunn@bristol.ac.uk*
Presented December 2015

Childbed fever is one of the oldest diseases known to man. It strikes women within hours or days of giving birth and has therefore been also called puerperal fever, or more recently puerperal sepsis. No disease, except perhaps for rickets, has had a greater impact on childbirth or on the fear with which it came to be regarded. I intend to trace the course of this disease over a period of two and a half thousand years using the observations and contributions of twelve doctors and one nurse as stepping stones in the rise and subsequent fall of this scourge of reproduction.

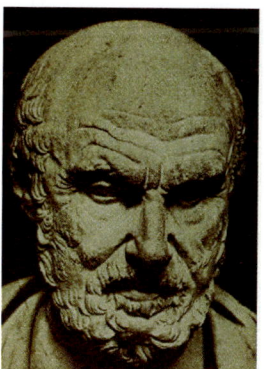

*Fig 1
Hippocrates (460-c356BC).*

As is so often the case we must reach back to Hippocrates of Cos (406-356BC) for our first stepping stone (Fig 1).

Hippocrates lived some 400 years before Christ. He was the first to mention childbed fever, writing:

'*Erysipelas attacking the internal surface of the pregnant uterus is destructive.*' [1]

As we shall see it is especially interesting that he used the term erysipelas.

400 years later Soranus of Ephesus (c AD 98-138) (Fig 2) provided a more complete clinical picture of puerperal inflammation of the uterus:

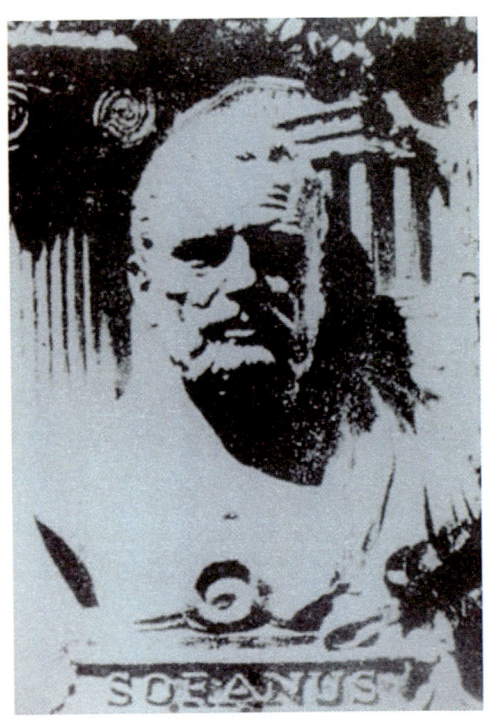

Fig 2.
Soranus of Ephesus (c AD 98-138)

'*The general signs which appear are the following: fever, furthermore pain and pulsation of the affected part, swelling and (rigidity), heat and dryness of the abdomen, tense feeling in the hips or heaviness in the loins, flanks, lower abdomen, groins and thighs, spells of shivering, a stabbing sensation, numbness of the feet and coldness of the knees, profuse perspiration, a small and very rapid pulse, sympathetic affection of the stomach, fainting, and weakness ... If the inflammation becomes worse, fever and swelling of the abdomen increase, delirium sets in as well as gnashing of the teeth (and) convulsions.'* [2]

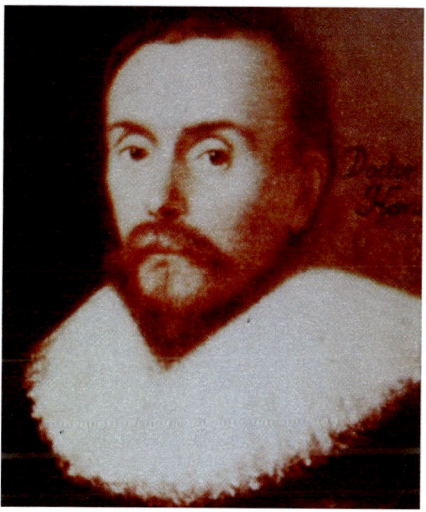

Fig 3
Dr. William Harvey (1578-1657)

The next significant contribution came with the Renaissance 1500 years later. The famous William Harvey (1578-1657) (Fig 3) wrote in 1650:
'It often happens especially in delicate women, that foul and putrid lochia set up fevers and other violent symptoms. Because the uterus, torn and injured by the separation of the placenta, especially if any violence has been used, resembles a vast internal ulcer, and is cleansed and purified by the free discharge of the lochia. Therefore, we do conclude as to the favourable or unfavourable state of the puerperal woman from the character of these secretions.' [3]

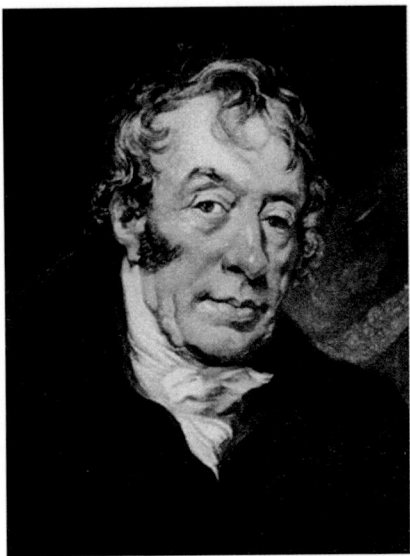

Fig 4
Charles White of Manchester (1728-1813).

In 1773 the great obstetrician, Charles White of Manchester (1728-1813) (Fig 4), recognised that childbed fever was contagious and that there was a need to isolate affected patients and to disinfect their rooms and bedding after use. Above all, he stressed the importance of prevention of the disease by strict cleanliness, good ventilation, and the encouragement of free drainage of the lochia by nursing the post-partum mother in a sitting position, and by early ambulation. After 21 years in practice, and at a time when one in 25 parturient women were dying from puerperal sepsis, he was able to claim that he had never lost a patient from this disease [4].

In the 18th and 19th centuries women, especially the poor, were increasingly delivered in hospital and the occurrence of epidemics of puerperal fever increased dramatically.

In 1795 the contagiousness of puerperal sepsis was emphasised by Alexander Gordon of Aberdeen (1752-1799). That city had

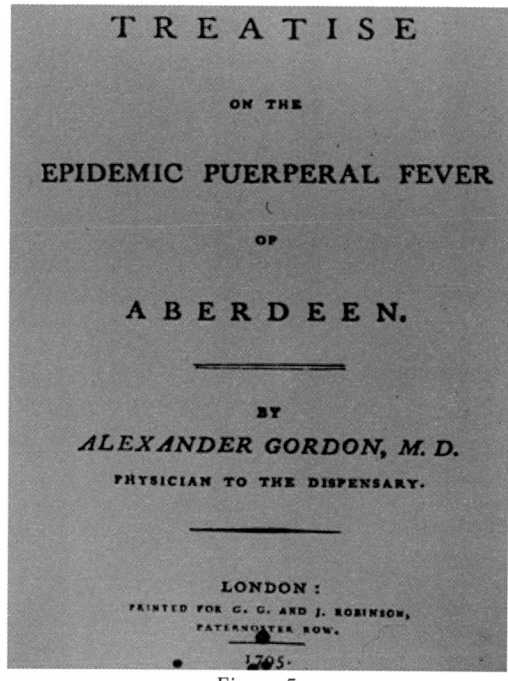

Figure 5
Frontpiece to Alexander Gordon's Treatise in 1795.

experienced two serious epidemics in 1789 and 1792 (Fig 5). He wrote:

'... *the cause of the epidemic puerperal fever is not owing to a noxious constitution of the atmosphere ... but this disease seizes such women only as were visited, or delivered, by a practitioner or taken care of by a nurse who had previously attended patients affected with the disease. In short, I had evident proof of its infectious nature, and that the infection was as readily communicated as that of the smallpox or measles, and operated more speedily than any other infection with which I am acquainted.*' [5]

Gordon also emphasised the relationship between erysipelas and puerperal sepsis, writing:

'*The analogy of the puerperal fever with erysipelas will explain why it always seized women after and not before delivery. For at the time when erysipelas was epidemic, almost every person admitted into our hospital with a wound, was, soon after his admission, seized with erysipelas in the vicinity of the wound.'* [5]

He added that:

'The patient's apparel and bedclothes ought to be burnt or thoroughly purified; and the nurses and physicians who have attended patients affected with the puerperal fever, ought carefully to wash themselves and to get their apparel properly fumigated before it be put on again.' [5]

The discovery of chlorine in 1774 had led gradually to its use as a disinfectant both of the hands as well as of the hospital wards and post-mortem rooms. In the 1830s, Robert Collins, master of the Rotunda Hospital, Dublin, (Fig 6) described how he terminated a series of epidemics of puerperal sepsis in his Hospital. After

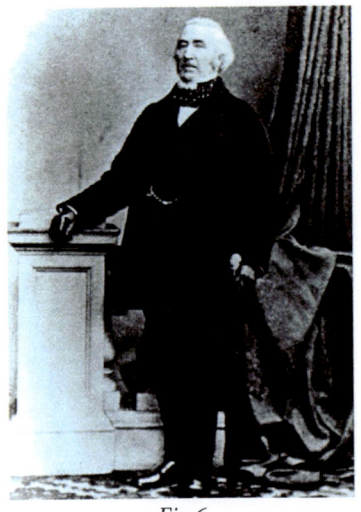

Fig 6
Robert Collins, Master of the Rotunda Hospital in Dublin (1826-1833).

temporary closure of the hospital, its contents were thoroughly cleansed and then fumigated with chlorine. Thereafter similar treatment was repeated ward by ward in rotation every ten to

twelve days. He reported in 1835 that in the last four years of his mastership:
'We did not lose one patient by this disease among 10,785 deliveries.' (6)
Following Collins' retirement as Master, the use of chlorine was discontinued and within a short time there was another serious epidemic of puerperal fever.
Meanwhile in the crowded public hospitals of Paris, London, Vienna and other large cities the ravages of puerperal fever were extremely severe.
In 1843 Dr. Oliver Wendell Holmes of Boston (1809-1894) (Fig 7), although not himself an obstetrician, convincingly marshalled the evidence demonstrating again that puerperal fever was contagious and was often spread between patients by their medical attendants.
He concluded his thesis with a series of pertinent recommendations on how to prevent the disease, ending with

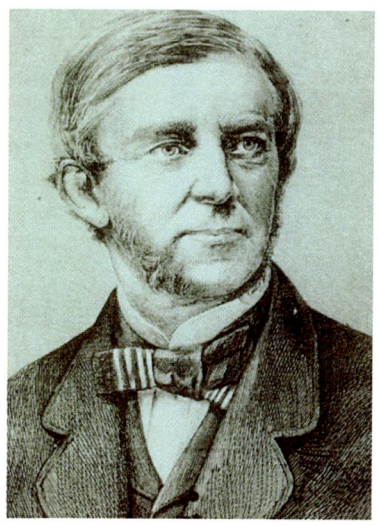

Fig 7
Oliver Wendell Holmes of Boston (1809-1894)

the following exhortation:

'Whatever indulgence may be granted to those who have heretofore been the ignorant causes of so much misery, the time has come when the existence of a private pestilence in the sphere of a single physician should be looked upon not as a misfortune but as a crime.' [7]

Yet, in spite of his plea, there were still many in Europe and America who for another twenty-five years or more, refused to accept the evidence. Thus, Professor Charles Meigs of Philadelphia wrote in 1848:

'Having practiced midwifery a great many years and having been concerned in the visitation of the sick labouring under puerperal fever ... visiting the same cases with those who have been so cruelly abused, as performing the part of a walking pestilence, scattering death and desolation where they desired only to do good – and seeing that I could never convict myself of being the means of spreading the contagion, I remain incredulous as to the contagiousness of the malady'. [8]

At much the same time as Holmes published his thesis, a young Hungarian obstetrician, Ignac Semmelweis (1818-1865) (Fig 8), was undertaking his own observations in the Vienna Krankhenhaus, where at that time one in seven delivered women were dying of puerperal fever. He, like Armstrong and Holmes before him, drew attention to the death from erysipelas and blood poisoning of doctors who had cut themselves while undertaking post-mortems on women dying of puerperal sepsis. His observations led him to similar conclusions to those of Armstrong and Holmes both as to cause and prevention. Although he spoke of his findings in 1850, because of illness (he contracted syphilis and departed hastily to Budapest) he did not actually publish his work until 1861[9,10].

In it he described the guilt he felt at having himself spread this fatal disease. He wrote:

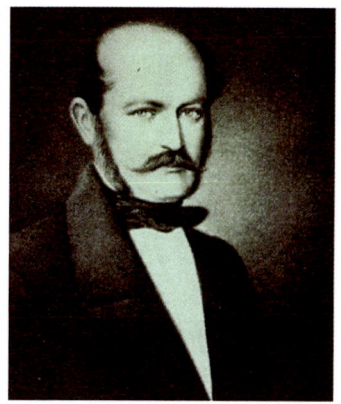
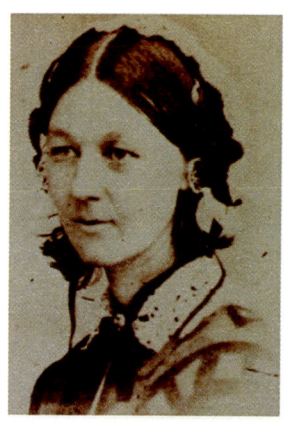

Fig 8
Professor Ignaz Semmelweis
(1818-1865).

Fig 9
Florence Nightingale
(1820-1910).

'Early (each) morning I conducted my gynaecological studies in the morgue. I then went to the labour room and began to examine all the patients, as I was obliged to do, so that I could report on each patient during the professor's morning rounds. My hands, contaminated by cadaverous particles, were thereby brought into contact with the genitals of many women in labour ... In consequence of my conviction I must affirm that only God knows the number of patients who went prematurely to their graves because of me.'[9,10]

Shortly after Semmelweis's report, which incidentally aroused a storm of protest and disbelief from many obstetricians throughout Europe, Florence Nightingale (1820-1910), famed for her work during the Crimean War, (Fig 9) was invited in 1867 to investigate an outbreak of puerperal sepsis at Kings College Hospital. In 1871 she reported her findings which included a list of the risk factors for puerperal fever and also the means of prevention [11].

'In future lying-in establishments should be well situated and isolated from any general hospital or medical school; the wards should be small and constantly rotated in use; they should

be frequently cleaned with lime washing; deliveries should be conducted by midwives specially attached to the labour wards; whenever possible the same birth attendant should look after mother and baby throughout; there should be early home discharge of the mothers; cases of puerperal fever should be immediately isolated; and there should be a reduction of intercommunication between lying-in and hospital divisions in terms of medical officers and nurses.' [11]

Between the 1850s and 1870s the discoveries of Louis Pasteur of France (1822-1897) (Fig 10), and Joseph Lister (1827-1912) in the UK (Fig 11) threw light on the bacterial nature of many

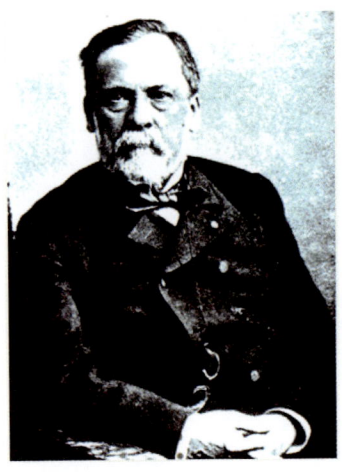
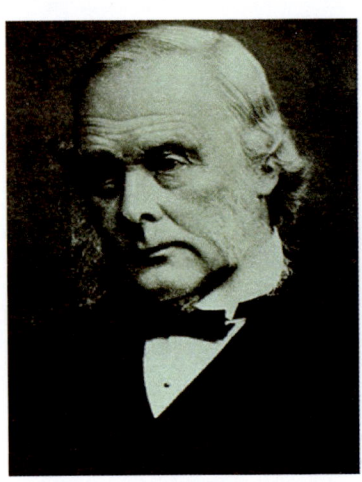

Fig 10
Louis Pasteur of Paris (1822-1897).

Fig 11
Lord Joseph Lister (1827-1912).

diseases, including wound sepsis and puerperal infection and also on the means of prevention, using first antisepsis with the carbolic acid spray and later an aseptic approach. Yet Lister's attempts to achieve antisepsis in surgical operating rooms met fierce opposition for many years both from administrators, physicians and surgeons who still disbelieved the germ theory of infection. However, the work of bacteriologists such as Robert

Koch of Germany (1843-1919) slowly won the day and it was Pasteur himself who in 1879 finally identified the beta-haemolytic streptococcus as the organism mainly responsible for puerperal fever [12].

In spite of these advances, including the use of heat sterilisation of instruments and the introduction of rubber gloves, puerperal fever continued to be a problem in maternity hospitals for several decades to come.

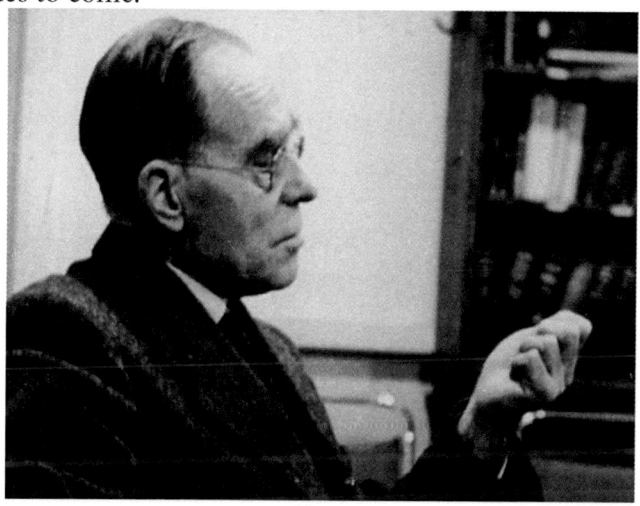

Fig 12
Dr. Leonard Colebrook 1883-1967).

Only with the advent of chemotherapy and then antibiotics was this scourge of childbirth finally defeated. In 1935 Professor Dogmagk of Germany introduced the bacterio-static drug prontosil and within a year Dr. Leonard Colebrook (1883-1967) (Fig 12) had demonstrated in the UK the remarkable effectiveness of both this drug and its derivative, sulphonamide, in the treatment of puerperal fever [13].

Meanwhile the bacteriologist, Alexander Fleming (1881-1955) (Fig 13), had observed in 1928 a stray mould, penicillium rubens, growing on a plate of bacteria. Around the mould

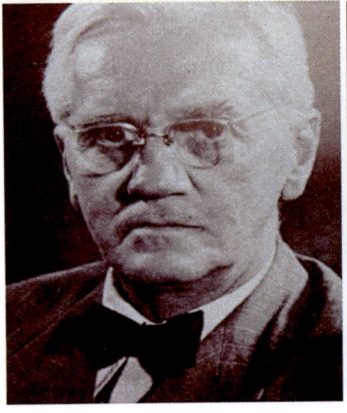
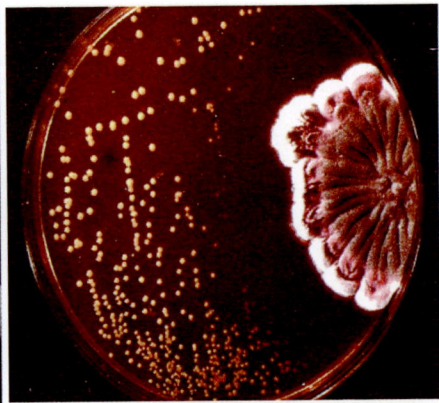

Fig 13
Sir Alexander Fleming
(1881-1955).

Fig 14
A culture of Fleming's penicillium notation demonstrating the inhibition of bacterial growth.

was a clear area where the bacteria had been killed (Fig 14). He recognised the significance of this observation and attempted without success to purify this bactericidal substance which he named penicillin[14.] It remained for Howard Florey (1898-1968) (Fig 15) and Ernest Chain working in Oxford to succeed in the production of penicillin in 1941 where Fleming had failed.

This antibiotic was introduced into the treatment of puerperal sepsis in 1945. The success of the sulphonamides and subsequently of penicillin in combating puerperal sepsis was reflected in the

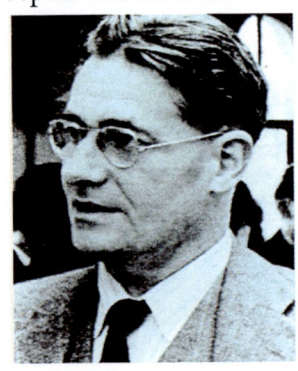

Fig 15
Baron Howard Florey (1898-1968).

falling maternal mortality figures for England and Wales that you see in this graph (Fig 16).

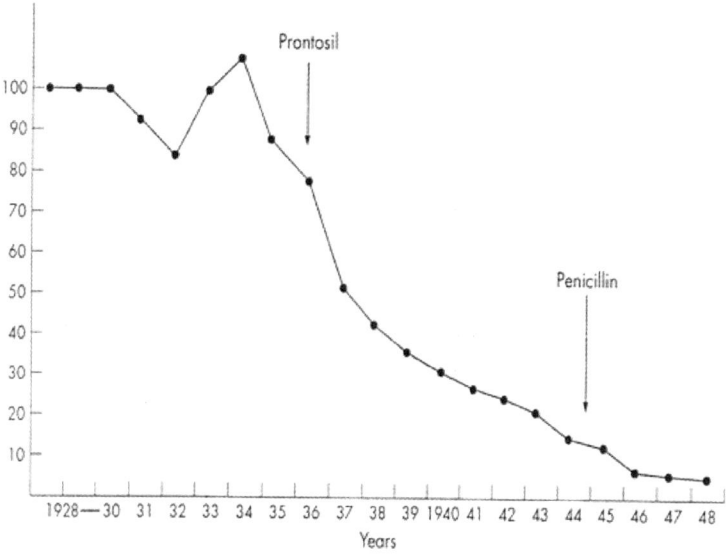

Fig 16
Puerperal sepsis mortality in England and Wales, 1928-30 is taken as 100 and the total for each subsequent year expressed in terms of that.

This account of the rise and the eventual fall of childbed fever over the years reveals how often the brilliant observations of certain doctors were either ignored, neglected or even opposed by their colleagues. The story emphasises the importance of and the need for doctors to have a knowledge of medical history.

REFERENCES

1. Adams. The genuine works of Hippocrates. London: the Sydenham Society, 1849.
2. Sorannus' Gynecology. Transl. by O. Tempkin. Baltimore: The John Hopkins Press, 1956
3. Harvey, W. The works of William Harvey. Transl. from Latin by R. Willis. London, the Sydenham Society, 1847; 1-624.
4. White, C. A treatise on the management of pregnant and lying-in women. London: Edward and Charles Dilly, 1773.
5. Gordon, A. A treatise on the epidemic puerperal fever of Aberdeen. London: G.G. and J. Robinson, 1795.
6. Collins, R. Practical treatise on midwifery containing the results of 16,654 births, occurring in the Dublin Lying-in Hospital during a period of seven years, commencing in November 1826. London: Longman et al, 1835.
7. Holmes, O.W. The contagiousness of puerperal fever. New Engl. Quart. J. Med. Surg., 1843, 1, 503-30.
8. Meigs, C.D. Obstetrics: the science and the art. Philadelphia: Lea and Blanchard, 1850.
9. Semmelweis, I. Die aetiology, der begriff, und die prophylaxis des kindbettfiebers. Pest, Wien u Leipzig: C.A. Hartleben, 1861.
10. Dunn, P.M. Ignac Semmelweis (1818-1865) of Budapest and the prevention of puerperal fever. Arch. Dis. Child. Fetal Neonatal Ed., 2005; 90, F345-F348.
11. Nightingale, F. Introductory notes on lying-in institutions. London: Longmans, Green & Co., 1871.
12. Pasteur, L. Septicémie puerperale. Bull. Acad. Méd. Paris, 1879; 8, 271-274.
13. Colebrook, L. The story of puerperal fever, 1800-1950. Brit. Med. J., 1956; 1, 247-252.
14. Fleming, A. On the antibacterial action of cultures of a penicillium, with special reference to their use in the isolation of B. Influenza. Brit. J. Experimental Pathology, 1929; 10, 226-236.

The Pill and the Pope

THOMAS F. BASKETT
MB, FRCS(C), FRCS (Ed), FRCOG, DHMSA
Emeritus Professor
Department of Obstetrics and Gynaecology
Dalhousie University
Halifax, Nova Scotia, Canada
Presented at the joint meeting with the
Bristol Medico Chirurgical Society April 2016

ABSTRACT

This talk outlines the development of the oral contraceptive pill and the roles of the individuals involved. Two formidable women, Margaret Sanger and Katherine McCormick, were the instigators and facilitators; Gregory Pincus, Min Chang, Russell Marker, Carl Djerassi and Frank Colton the scientists and John Rock, Celso Garcia and Edris Rice-Wray the clinicians. Their contribution to the development of the pill and the early evolution of the birth control movement will be outlined.

The pill stimulated the Catholic Church to confront its position on contraception, and in 1963 the Pontifical Commission on Birth Control was established to advise the Pope. The recommendations of the commission and the Pope's response will be discussed.

MARGARET SANGER

Margaret Sanger (1879 – 1966) was the most influential person in the campaign for women's sexual and reproductive freedom in North America during the first half of the 20th century. She was born Margaret Higgins to Irish immigrant parents from

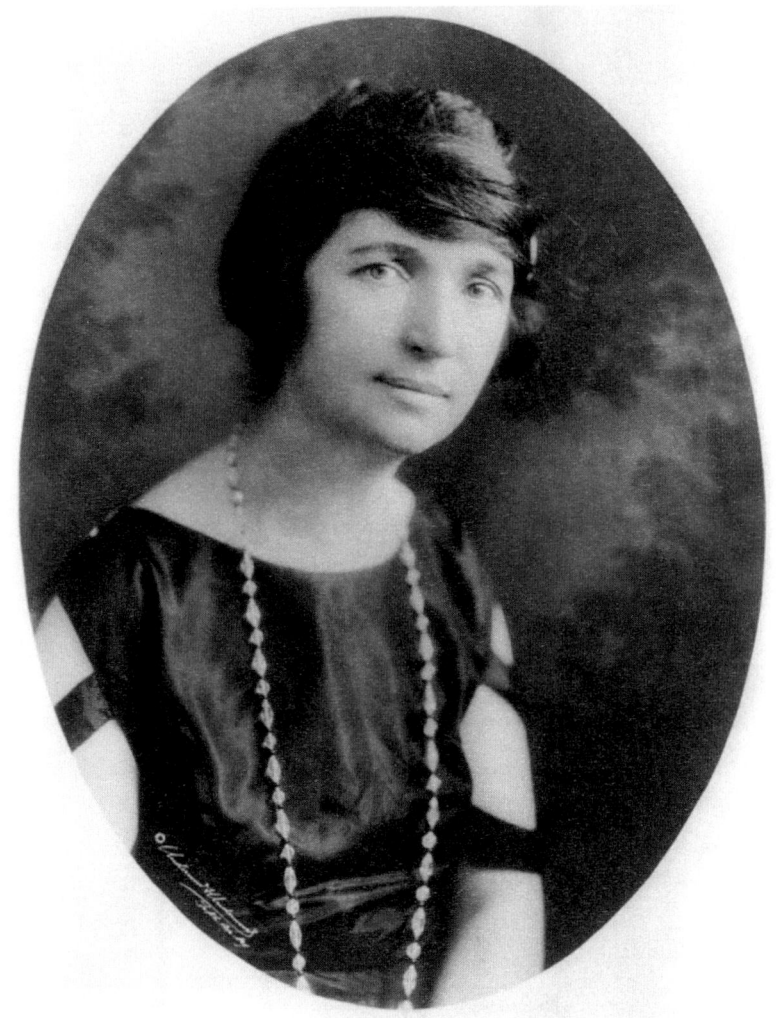

Margaret Sanger

Cork and, as the sixth of eleven children, was raised in modest circumstances in Corning, New York. After training as a nurse she married William Sanger, an architect and artist, had three children and for a time lived as a mother and housewife. This changed in 1911 when the family moved to Greenwich Village,

New York and both she and her husband embraced socialism and women's rights. For two years she was employed as a nurse by the New York Social Welfare Agency, working among the tenements of the very poor, mostly immigrant families. Sanger was struck by the crippling poverty associated with unlimited reproduction and by the total ignorance of all methods of contraception, except for the $5.00 back street abortion. In 1913 she stopped nursing and committed herself to the promotion of women's sexual and reproductive rights. She visited France and was impressed by the sophistication and the knowledge of sex and contraception of French women. Upon return to New York she started a newsletter, The Woman Rebel, in which she coined the term 'birth control' and encouraged women to *"Look the whole world in the face with a go-to-hell look in the eyes"*. The monthly newsletter only lasted from March to October 1914 before she was indicted under the Comstock Law.

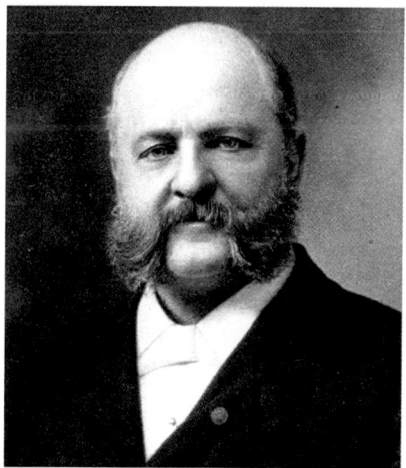

Anthony Comstock

Anthony Comstock (1844 – 1915) was president of the Society for the Suppression of Vice – a committee of the Young Men's Christian Association (YMCA). In this capacity he collected available pornographic material and used this to lobby congress to abolish the distribution of such material, including information on contraception, under a new law – which he helped draft. The so-called Comstock Law prohibited "Obscene, lewd or lascivious material. All devices or information preventing conception," and remained on the books from 1873 to 1971.

Margaret Sanger, realising she did not have the profile or support necessary to fight the charge, fled to Britain via train to Montreal and thence by ship to Liverpool. There she connected with birth control and sexual liberation advocates and practiced the principles of both movements. A year later, in September 1915, she had to return to New York to look after her children when her husband was jailed for distributing some of her birth control leaflets. Due to the intervention of some influential British advocates, including Marie Stopes and HG Wells, the former charges against her were dropped. She focused her efforts on birth control education and helped found the National Birth Control League in the United States – the forerunner of Planned Parenthood. In October 1916 she opened the first birth control clinic in America, in the same poor area of New York in which she had worked as a nurse; there were > 100 patient visits on the first day. Within days, as she anticipated, the clinic was shut down by the police as she once again fell foul of the Comstock Law. Her trial attracted a lot of publicity, she conducted her own defence and was sentenced to 30 days in prison. After this, as she had planned, her public profile was assured and she used this podium to embark upon extensive speaking tours. In particular, she railed against the Catholic church's position on contraception: *"Church control or birth control.....The dictatorship of celibates"*.
In 1920, on her initiative, she divorced William Sanger. She told her sister she needed to find a rich husband to fund her cause. This she did, in the form of James Noah Slee, the founder

and president of Three-in-One oil. This enabled her to fund her activities in the promotion of birth control including her speaking tours, literature, conferences and support for Planned Parenthood. She retained the name Sanger, as this was linked to her public persona.

Like many who fight against accepted dogma Margaret Sanger was egotistical, single-minded and relentless. She sent her young children to boarding schools and focused her efforts entirely on the birth control movement, which she regarded as her cause. Initially she embraced the eugenics movement, but later tried to distance herself from their teachings. She was promiscuous, manipulative and often fought with others – even those who shared her views on birth control. Showing some insight into her own character she once said, *"I am not a fit person for love, home, children, friends or anything which needs attention or consideration."* Be that as it may, no one in the first half of the 20th century matched her sustained and effective commitment, for more than 50 years, to the cause of women's freedom over their own sexuality and reproduction – culminating, as we shall see, in the development of the oral contraceptive pill.

KATHERINE McCORMICK

Katherine McCormick (1875 – 1967) was the other main protagonist in the instigation and development of the pill. She was born Katherine Dexter, into a rich and prominent legal family in Chicago. In 1904, she was the first woman to graduate with a science degree (biology) from the Massachusetts Institute of Technology. Shortly after graduation she married Stanley McCormick, the son and heir to the extensive McCormick farm machine business. Sadly, within a year of the marriage, Stanley McCormick descended into dysfunctional madness, said to be a type of schizophrenia, from which he never recovered. Extensive

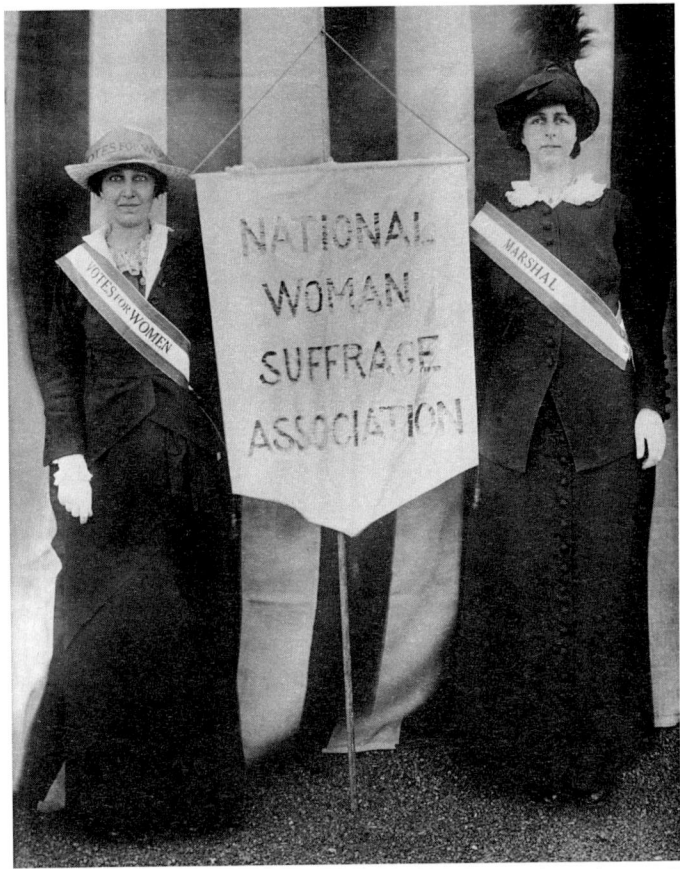

Suffragists Mrs. Stanley McCormick (Katharine McCormick) and Mrs. Charles Parker, April 22, 1913, holding a banner between them reading "National Woman Suffrage Association."

private treatment and funding of neuro-psychiatric research was of no avail and he died in 1944. Katherine McCormick ultimately inherited both her family and the McCormick estates, making her exceptionally rich. She helped fund the Woman's Suffrage movement and participated in their demonstrations. Through her support of Planned Parenthood she came in contact with Margaret Sanger and they forged a friendship based on their common support of women's reproductive rights.

Gregory Pincus (1903 – 1967) was the son of Russian parents who fled the anti-semitic pogroms in Odessa and settled in New Jersey. He was brought up on a collective farm there and entered Cornell University, gaining degrees in biology. In 1931 he was appointed assistant professor at Harvard University, where he became an expert on mammalian reproduction. This included creating a rabbit embryo by fertilising a rabbit egg and sperm in a petri dish – the forerunner of in vitro fertilisation. Which feat gained him considerable publicity – not all of it favourable. His time at Harvard included a sabbatical leave for one year at Cambridge University. At the end of his seven year appointment at Harvard Pincus was denied tenure. He therefore took up a relatively minor appointment in the department of physiology at Clark University, Worcester – a town some 50 miles west of Boston. In 1944, frustrated by a lack of time and resources for research, Pincus and a former Harvard colleague, Hudson Hoagland, founded the Worcester Foundation for Experimental Biology – based, in fact, in the adjacent town of Shrewsbury. This was an audacious move that involved buying and converting a large house and small estate – in part funded by donations they solicited from local business and citizens. At this time the chemical structure of human hormones was being refined and there was great interest in steroid chemistry in general. In particular, the medical use of sex hormones, cortisone and allied compounds was increasing. As a result government agencies and the pharmaceutical industry required extensive animal testing on various promising compounds. Such contracts enabled Pincus and Hoagland to get their new foundation established. Pincus was very bright, driven and blessed with a photographic memory; his core belief was *"In science everything is possible"*.

By late 1951 both Sanger and McCormick were disillusioned with the direction of Planned Parenthood's research programmes.

They felt that a new contraceptive was needed; one that the woman controlled and was independent of each act of intercourse. In essence, they wanted a pill that the woman took to render her temporarily sterile. Sanger was familiar with Pincus' work having met him at scientific meetings. She and Katherine McCormick arranged to meet with Pincus at the Worcester Foundation and, after a preliminary tour and pleasantries, they got down to business. McCormick led the discussion: could Pincus develop an oral contraceptive pill? Pincus thought it was feasible. How much funding would he need to concentrate on this work? Pincus replied $125,000 (> $1million in current funds). McCormick wrote a cheque for $40,000 ($360,000) and told Pincus the remaining $85,000 ($765,000) would follow shortly. Over the next eight years, until the pill was approved in 1960, McCormick supported Pincus in the amount of $2 million ($15-18 million). No government agency or pharmaceutical company would fund the research because of the many state laws forbidding contraception. At the time of this meeting Sanger was 73 years old and McCormick was 77. Sanger was frail, having had repeated heart attacks. She retired to Arizona and, fueled by champagne and pethidine, withdrew from active participation in the project; other than via correspondence. McCormick moved from California to Boston; periodically arriving at the Foundation in her chauffeur–driven Rolls Royce to receive progress reports and provide encouragement. *"Freezing in Boston for the pill"* as she put it.

Pincus got to work. He employed Min-Chueh Chang (1908-1991) a fellow scientist from China with whom he had worked in Cambridge. At this time the reproductive cycle and control of ovulation was understood. Their previous work and that of others showed that progesterone inhibited ovulation in animals. However, the source of progesterone for study was from animal ovaries – which was scarce and very expensive; it took 25,000 sow ovaries to produce 1mg progesterone. For this reason laboratories that produced sex hormones were set up beside abattoirs. Fortunately, Russel Marker (1902-1995), by dint of brilliant chemistry and detective work found an abundant plant source of progesterone in the Mexican yam. The other drawback was that progesterone, to be fully active, had to be given by injection. This was solved by two scientists, Carl Djerassi (1923-2015) and Frank Colton (1923-2003) who produced orally active progestins: norethindrone and norethynodrel respectively – the latter was used in the first oral contraceptive pill.

By 1954 Pincus was ready to embark upon human trial and for this he sought the aid of a prominent Boston obstetrician/gynaecologist. John Rock (1890-1984) was the grandson of famine-era immigrants from Armagh, Northern Ireland, Harvard educated and with an interest in infertility. He was also a devout Catholic who attended mass every day. However, in his later years he had become very concerned about population control on a global scale. When Pincus approached him with his proposal for a contraceptive pill Rock said this could not be done in Massachusetts, which had the most restrictive state law against contraception. Rock was however already treating infertile women with progesterone for several months in the hope of getting a rebound fertility effect after stopping the progesterone. All his patients knew they could not get pregnant while they were taking progesterone. He agreed to use the Pincus pill on the same basis and make the required observations. This study confirmed that the progesterone pill did consistently suppress ovulation in humans as it had in animals.

The next step was to organise larger human trials which, because of the restrictive laws, could not be done in the United States.

Working with Rock at that time was the New York trained gynaecologist Celso Ramon Garcia (1922-2004), also a Catholic. He had previously worked in Puerto Rico and suggested it as a suitable setting for a trial, with a fertile Catholic population but no law against contraception. Pincus, Rock and Garcia visited Puerto Rico and were fortunate to find a willing local clinical co-ordinator in Edris Rice-Wray (1904-1990). She was an American trained doctor from Detroit and the Director of the Puerto Rico Family Planning Association. Garcia worked closely with her in conducting the trial. An additional trial was carried out in Haiti, under the supervision of Dr Felix Laraque. A serendipitous finding was that one batch of the progestin pill, subsequently shown to be contaminated with oestrogen, produced fewer side effects in the form of less breakthrough bleeding. Thus, the final pill was comprised of both progestin and a small amount of oestrogen. During the early development of the pill all pharmaceutical companies had refused to participate. G.D. Searle, a small company in Skokie, Illinois had funded some of Pincus' steroid research and they finally agreed to produce and market the pill as Enovid. Ultimately, Enovid was approved by the Food and Drug Administration (FDA) for gynaecological disorders in 1957 and as an oral contraceptive in 1960. The modern pill contains about one eighth the amount of hormones in Enovid.

THE CATHOLIC CHURCH

The position of the Catholic Church vis a vis contraception was straight forward – it was a grave sin. How this came to be is less clear to the outside observer. There was the exhortation in the book of Genesis to 'increase and multiply' and 'fill the earth', and notables such as St Augustine and St Thomas Aquinas condemned contraception as 'unlawful' and 'wicked'. However, within the church prohibition of contraception was doctrine, rather than written law. Indeed, there was no reference to contraception in the New Testament and the only possible inference in the Old Testament was Onan spilling his seed on the ground; the latter being more an act against Judaic law, with failure to carry on the family name. The first written papal ruling on the matter came in 1930 from Pope Pius XI (1922-39), and his encyclical Casti Connubii ('Of Chaste Marriage') in which he described contraception as "An offence against the law of God.....a grave sin.....and intrinsically vicious." This may have been in response to the Protestant church's relaxation of its ban on contraception at the 1930 Lambeth Conference of Bishops. In 1951, his successor, Pope Pius XII (1939-58) declared that "Observance of the natural sterile periods may be lawful from the moral standpoint" and that "The husband and wife may use their matrimonial right even during the days of natural sterility." The days of 'natural sterility' referred to the rhythm or safe period method of contraception – the only one acceptable to the Catholic church. This was the first time that the church acknowledged that sexual intercourse could be undertaken without the aim or likelihood of procreation.

Pope John XXIII (1958-63) established the Pontifical Commission on Population, Family and Birth in 1963 to advise him on birth control - stimulated in part by the development of the pill and its increasing acceptance by Catholic married couples. He also acknowledged the increasing global population – the 'demographic problem' as he put it. In the 50 years after his recognition of the problem, from 1960 to 2010, the world's population increased from 3 billion to 7 billion.

Pope Paul VI (1963-78) was to inherit the commission after the death of John XXIII. Early in his papacy he received a petition from 182 Catholic theological scholars urging him

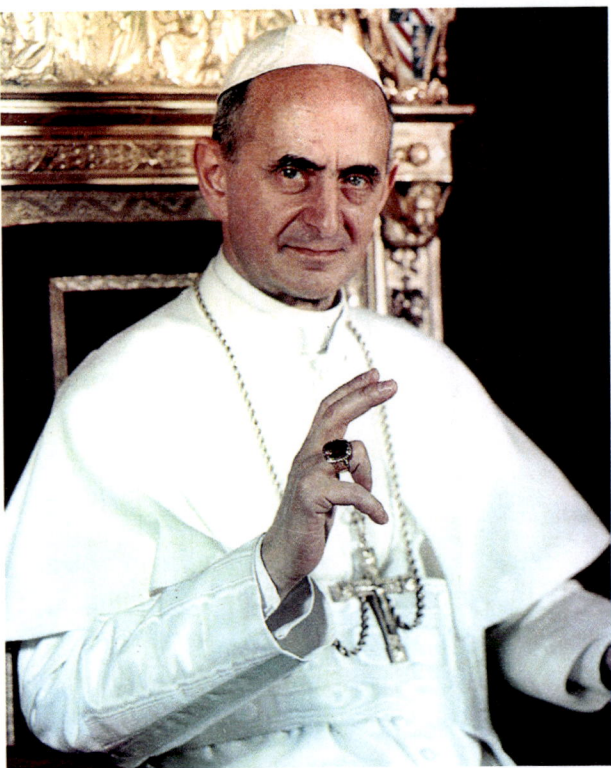
Pope Paul VI

to give a 'far-reaching reappraisal' of the church's position on contraception. A number of theologians argued in favour of the church changing its position on contraception in view of the widespread use of birth control methods by otherwise devout Catholic parishioners. Most felt it should be a matter of individual conscience. Pope Paul expanded the commission to 58 members and added an executive committee of 16 bishops, to be chaired by Cardinal Alfredo Ottaviani (1890-1979), who was Secretary of the Holy Office. The commission included three lay couples who presented a survey of members of the Christian Family Movement, outlining the impact on married couples of the church's teaching on contraception. The argument of those in favour of the church sanctioning the pill was that it did not interfere with sexual intercourse and that it acted by extending the 'natural sterile' periods of the woman's cycle. The commission presented its report to the Pope in 1966. The results were to be confidential but were leaked to a Catholic newsletter in the United States. A large majority of the commission's theologian/lay members and a smaller majority of the bishops supported change. The Pope took two years to formulate his response. During this time he was influenced by Cardinal Ottaviani, whose position could be summed up by his personal motto *Semper Idem ('Always the same')*. One of the considerations was that Popes were infallible and spoke eternal truths. Thus, if Pope Paul changed the church's position on contraception, the inference could be that his predecessors were, in fact, fallible and that eternal truths were not so eternal.

On 25 July, 1968 Pope Paul issued his encyclical Humanae Vitae ('Of Human Life') which reaffirmed Catholic teachings: " The church…..condemns as always unlawful the use of means which directly prevent conception, even when the reasons given for the latter practice may appear to be upright and serious".
In the end the Pope did not take the commission's advice and was more concerned with how change might affect the authority of the church rather that the effect on the church's flock. Even though the Second Vatican Council had reaffirmed, in 1965, that the church was the flock and not the hierarchy. Unsurprisingly, the encyclical was greeted with widespread disbelief and condemnation by laity and priests across Europe, Scandinavia and North America. In general, educated Catholics and many priests continued to ignore this component of the church's teaching. Thus, the credibility and authority of the Pope was undermined – the opposite of Pope Paul's rationale for continuing the church's contraception dogma.

John Rock became the most credible and prominent spokesman for birth control in the years following the pill's launch. He was profoundly disappointed in Pope Paul's encyclical and hoped that a subsequent pope would soften the church's stance on contraception. It was not to be, and the three successors to Pope Paul have only confirmed his 1968 encyclical. Surveys consistently show that the vast majority of the Catholic laity and priests do not believe that contraception is immoral. In a sense the church's authorities have painted themselves into a corner by citing papal infallibility and eternal truths over the past century.

BIBLIOGRAPHY

1. Asbell B. The Pill: A Biography of the Drug that Changed the World. New York: Random House; 1995.

2. Baskett TF. On the Shoulders of Giants: Eponyms and Names in Obstetrics and Gynaecology. Cambridge: Cambridge University Press; 2008.

3. Burns J. The American Rebellion Against Humanae Vitae. 2011.

4. Djerassi C. The Politics of Contraception. New York: WW Norton & Co; 1979.

5. Eig J. The Birth of the Pill. New York: WW Norton & Co; 2014.

6. Fryer P. The Birth Controllers. New York: Stein and Day; 1966.

7. Langley LL (ed). Benchmark Papers in Human Physiology: Contraception. Straudsberg: Dowden, Hutchinson & Ross, Inc; 1973.

8. Marks LV. Sexual Chemistry: A History of the Contraceptive Pill. New Haven: Yale University Press: 2010.

9. May ET. America and the Pill. New York: Basic Books; 2010.

10. McLaughlin L. The Pill, John Rock and the Church: the Biography of a Revolution. Boston: Little Brown Co; 1982.

11. Rock J. The Time Has Come. London: Catholic Book Club;1963.

12. Speroff L. A Good Man: Gregory Goodwin Pincus. Portland: Amica Publishing, Inc; 2009.

13. Tentler LW. Catholics and Contraception: An American History. Ithaca: Cornell University Press: 2004.

14. Wood C, Suitters B. The Fight for Acceptance: A History of Contraception. Aylesbury: Medical and Technical Publishing Co Ltd; 1970.

Unhealthy Bristol -
Just how bad were conditions in the 1840s?

PETER MALPASS
Emeritus Professor of Housing Policy and Head of the School of Housing and
Urban Studies at the University of the West of England, Bristol
Presented June 2016

The rapid growth in the urban population as a whole in the first four decades of the 19th Century was accompanied by an alarming decline in the quality of life in the very towns that were propelling Britain towards domination of the global economy. As people poured into towns to live and work rivers and streams became heavily polluted by both domestic and industrial waste, supplies of well water became tainted, accumulations of filth were everywhere and a resurgence of infectious diseases, especially among the poorest and most overcrowded sections of the population, reduced life expectancy. Epidemics of cholera (the first in 1831-2) caused panic in the short term, but far more deaths resulted from endemic diseases such as typhus and tuberculosis. The Victorian concern with sanitation and public health began to crystallise in 1838 when three reports written for the Poor Law Commissioners by Doctors Neil Arnott, James Kay and Thomas Southwood Smith *'most emphatically fixed the blame for the spread of disease on squalid urban conditions'*.[1] Population growth placed heavy demands on the existing urban infrastructure, specifically the supply of housing and established methods of supplying water and disposing of sewage and refuse. Appropriate responses were slow to emerge. It has been asserted by Professor Flinn that, *'Most of the more intransigent social problems of this period grew out of the ever-increasing concentration of the population in towns'*.[2] However, this requires to be qualified by recognition that problems arose not from the size or density of urban populations as such but from their relation to the systems in place to deal with people's needs. There were two sides to the problem: first, the sheer number of people required a commensurate increase in housing supply and a step change in the way water was supplied and waste removed, and second, the rate of population increase was such that conditions became much worse before the necessary changes were devised and implemented.

Although Bristol was spared the extraordinary increases experienced in some places its population doubled between 1801 and 1841, and in 1845 it was revealed to be among the least healthy of all large towns. Indeed, the claim was later made that mortality in Bristol 'was exceeded by only two towns in the kingdom'.[3] This was an alarmist and exaggerated misinterpretation of limited evidence, but there is no doubt that Bristol was a very dirty, smelly and unhealthy place to live.

The story to be told in this paper concerns the revelation of the dreadful environmental conditions endured by people (especially, but not exclusively, the poor) in Bristol in the 1840s. Reform of local government in Bristol in the 1830s was initiated by central government, and the same was true of public health in the 1840s. The reason that we have detailed accounts of the health and living conditions of the people of Bristol at that time is entirely due to the emergence of a national movement for public health reform and the initial momentum given to it by the reports of Doctors Arnott, Kay and Southwood Smith, and by the leadership provided by Edwin Chadwick, *'who saw the transformation of the environment through state action as the key to both health and prosperity'*.[4]

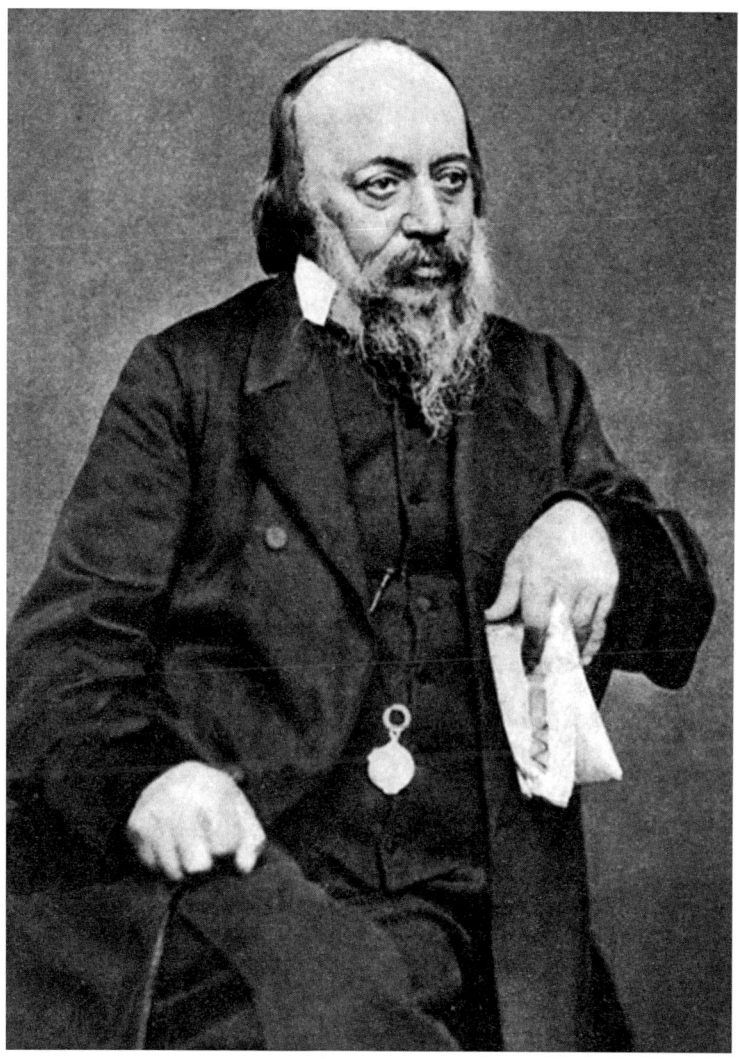

Sir Edwin Chadwick

Chadwick was the secretary to the Poor Law Commission from 1834 to 1842, but he had a difficult relationship with his employers, who were happy to give him leave of absence from 1839 to work on what became his Report on the Sanitary

Condition of the Labouring Population of Great Britain (1842). The revelations set out in this *'magisterial, comprehensive and horrendous indictment of social conditions in Britain'*[5] were not sufficient to prompt immediate policy action, but in 1843 a Royal Commission was appointed to look into the state of large towns and populous districts (often referred to as the health of towns commission).

Chadwick was not a member of the commission but he nevertheless drafted most of its first report in 1844.[6] This time there was a legislative response, albeit delayed until passage of the Public Health Act, 1848, which was the first piece of national legislation on the problem. Whereas the 1842 report had nothing to say about Bristol, the royal commission generated two investigations into conditions in the city, and as a consequence of the 1848 Act a third empirical survey was carried out, in 1850. These reports provide a rich source of evidence on just how awful were the conditions in Bristol in the 1840s, but it is important to remember that they were written for effect, to strengthen the case for reform, and therefore they should not be seen as entirely objective analyses. Nevertheless, reading them today it is impossible not to be impressed by the sheer weight of descriptive and statistical evidence.

In 1843 Dr William Kay was asked to write a report on the sanitary condition of Clifton for the health of towns commission.[7] As the senior physician at the Clifton Dispensary he was in a good position to combine detailed first hand observations with carefully constructed statistical tables of morbidity and mortality.[8] His report, completed in January 1844, vividly describes not only the foul dwellings of the poor living along Hotwell Road, close to the floating harbour, but also draws attention to the grossly offensive smells encountered in parts of upper Clifton. He refers, for example, to a surface drain at the top of Granby Hill which *'assails the olfactories'*, and another one, equally offensive,

on Clifton Hill. But it was in lower Clifton (Hotwells) that he encountered the worst housing conditions. At one house above the floating harbour Kay visited a sick patient:
'Upon entering the room, a smell of the most foul and offensive nature, and which, on so elevated a site, I was little prepared to encounter, betrayed the secret mischief. I presently discovered that a door, close to the head of the patient's bed, communicated directly with the pig-stye [sic]; anything more disgustingly loathsome than the intolerable stench which escaped from the mingled odours of wash [ie pigswill] and excrement, it is impossible to conceive.'
The housing (and slaughtering) of animals in such close proximity to people was not unusual at the time, and Kay went on to note that although the man died the pigs remained. Smell was a constant theme in the reports of reformers such as William Kay, not only because bad smells were in themselves repellent but also because they were seen as the cause of illness. The importance of ventilation was therefore another recurrent theme.

Kay drew attention to Rees's Court (off Hotwell Road) as an overcrowded and ill-ventilated place with a particularly high incidence of typhus and other infectious diseases. Just along the street was Jones's Court, where sixteen houses accommodating 116 people surrounded two open spaces only 8ft 6 inches and 9ft 6 inches wide respectively. Unsurprisingly Kay found this to be ill-ventilated, dirty and badly drained. Some commentators were inclined to blame the residents for the foul and dirty conditions, but Kay was adamant that the true causes were defective drainage, imperfect ventialtion, crowded and badly constructed dwellings and absence of a proper water supply.

William Kay's report was drawn on by the two members of the health of towns commission, Sir Henry de la Beche and Dr Lyon Playfair who carried out their own investigation in Bristol. Their report, published in 1845,[9] contained accounts of their observations as well as evidence submitted to them by informed

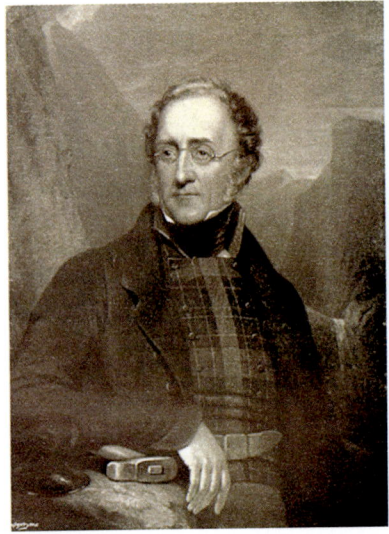 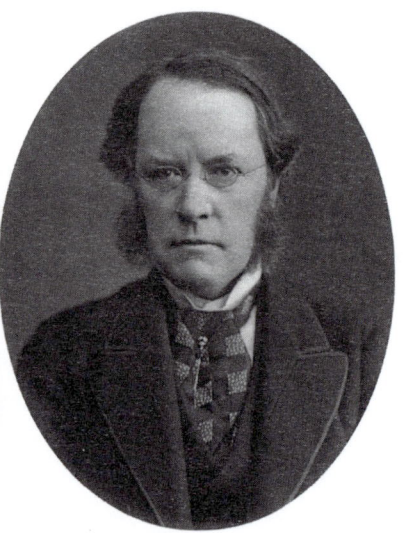

Sir Henry de la Beche and Dr Lyon Playfair

local witnesses, including doctors such as William Budd and clergymen with city centre parishes. A measure of both the awfulness of the task confronting the two commissioners, and their commitment to gathering evidence, is the account (provided by Edwin Chadwick himself) of how de la Beche '*was obliged to stand up at the end of alleys and vomit while Dr Playfair was inspecting overflowing privies*'.[10] Their report amounted to a serious indictment of the conditions endured by the people of Bristol, especially those living in the poorer, lower lying areas nearest to the two rivers, in particular the Frome. This small river was described as the '*chief sewage nuisance of Bristol*' as it wound its way through the town before reaching the floating harbour. In dry weather the flow of water became little more than a trickle, not enough to cover the waste draining or being thrown into it, never mind wash it away. Only the poor would tolerate living next to it and the Lewin's Mead area was said to consist of wretched courts and tenements. Dr Budd's evidence referred to the '*noisome effluvia*' from the Frome. He went on to say that *'In many parts, the aspect of the ditch and its banks, loaded with impurities of all kinds, is disgusting in the extreme. Between St John's bridge and the bridge at the Quay-head the nuisance reaches its climax. The inhabitants of Christmas-street are the great sufferers'.*

De la Beche also pointed to the continuing nuisance represented by the floating harbour, into which a mass of sewage was still discharged despite the improvements carried out in the 1820s. Increases in population since that time must have made matters worse. It was later admitted that *'...during hot and dry seasons, the fetid vapours arising from [the floating harbour], are sufficient to prejudice seriously the health of the inhabitants residing in its vicinity'*.[11] The report was critical of the drainage and sewerage of the town as a whole, although it was recognised that the Paving and Lighting Commissioners were doing their best in difficult circumstances and with few resources. Part of the problem was that the Commissioners only had authority within the ancient city boundaries, but significant numbers of people then lived further out. *'A large portion of the sewerage of the out parish of St Philip and St Jacob is in a miserable state: there is one district, termed the Dings, in which it is wretched. It is also very bad in many parts of Bedminster'*. Even in the affluent parts of Clifton *'the want of proper sewerage is deplorable. Ranges of handsome houses, otherwise well appointed, have nothing but a system of cesspools – often holes from which the stones for building the chief and rough parts of the houses have been taken'*.

The problem of sewerage was intimately linked with that of water supply. Traditionally, the sewers were intended to be land drains, discharging into rivers and streams from which the people drew their water. They were therefore supposed to be kept clean and free of human and animal waste, and the Act of 1806 that created the Bristol Paving Commissioners specified penalties to be incurred by anyone depositing 'lime, clay rubbish or any other matter or thing' in the public sewers and drains. In practice, however, it was obvious to everyone that a good deal of foul waste was finding its way into the sewers and rivers, either because people simply dumped it there in defiance of the rules, or because of natural seepage from cesspools and middens. Before the general adoption of water borne sewerage waste matter from household privies was typically buried in the garden (where there was one) or stored in a cesspool, which would eventually require to be emptied. Needless to say, the emptying of cesspools was a deeply unpleasant business for all concerned, both the 'nightmen' whose job it was to shovel the stuff out, the people living in the house being cleansed and those living nearby. Privies were almost invariably placed outside but sometimes the nightmen had to carry buckets and tubs through the house itself before carting the stinking material away to a depot where it could be dried and sold for fertiliser – or simply left to accumulate.[12] However, there are references to the contents of cesspools being pumped out into the open street gutters.[13] Keeping privies anything like clean was a major problem, especially when water was scarce and had to be fetched by hand. The problem was made worse when privies were shared by numbers of families. De la Beche reported that in Bristol:

'A deficient supply of privies, occasionally in bad repair, and very often filthy, forms the only means of [sanitary] accommodation for the poorer classes. In some districts which we examined, we found as many as one privy for every two houses. In other districts, the proportion was three privies for 14 houses; and in several instances the supply was still more scanty. There are no regulations for cleansing privies, except an implied private understanding, that each of the neighbours enjoying the advantage shall cleanse them in rotation.'[14]

Each house in Bristol contained on average 6.1 people at that time, so in the worst cases there were probably thirty people per privy, and the Paving Commissioners had no powers to compel owners of houses to drain their properties into the public sewers. Cesspools were often constructed so that liquid content could drain or seep away, thereby extending the period between visits from the nightmen. However, effluent entering the subsoil could pollute the water in wells from which people drew their supplies. De la Beche reported that in some parts of Bristol little care was taken to prevent filth oozing into wells, and in the Dings area he had seen a privy immediately adjacent to a well. Inevitably as urban densities increased the risks of pollution in this way also increased, although the dangers inherent in drinking tainted water were not understood until after the discovery of the link between cholera and polluted water. The link was theorised by Dr John Snow in London in the late 1840s and proved by him during the cholera epidemic of 1854. However, doctors in Bristol, notably William Budd were thinking along similar lines, challenging the prevailing idea that disease was produced and spread by foul air.[15]

The water supply in Bristol was undeniably deficient. De la Beche noted that

'The...city of Bristol, containing, with Clifton, 130,000 inhabitants, is not supplied with water under the provisions of any Act of Parliament, and the supply is most inadequate, probably more so than than in any town of equal size in England.'[16]

People needed water for drinking and cooking, cleaning and washing, and of course a constant supply was a necessary precondition of the development of the sort of water borne sewerage that we take for granted. De la Beche concluded that *'It is probably considerably above the truth, that not more than 5,000 persons, and theses constituting the most wealthy families in Bristol and Clifton, are supplied with water by means of pipes laid on into their houses'.*[17] The great majority depended on wells and rain barrels. Dr Budd and others submitted evidence stating that the filthy conditions in which the Bristol poor survived was in large measure due to the lack of water rather than inherent habits of the people themselves.

In view of the evidence of overcrowding, poor ventialtion, deficient sanitation and inadequate water supply presented by William Kay and Henry de la Beche it is not surprising that Bristol suffered from high mortality. What is perhaps more surprising is that Bristol appeared to have one of the highest mortality rates in Britain, 'inferior only to Liverpool and Manchester' according to de la Beche. This has been repeated in numerous publications ever since and so it is important both to say that the evidence is not clearcut and to understand how the claim came to be made. Its origin seems to lie in the fourth annual report of the Registrar General, dated August 1842, which included a table showing the annual mortality in ten large towns averaged over the period 1838-40. Bristol was in fact the fourth, not third, worst of these ten, but there was no suggestion in the text that these were the places with the highest mortality rates. William Kay reproduced part of this table in his report, but left out Salford which had a higher mortality than Bristol, thereby allowing de la Beche to draw the conclusion that Bristol was the third most unhealthy place.

An interesting, and not insignificant, feature of the Registrar General's table (as reproduced by Kay) was that it presented separate figures for Bristol and Clifton. This was because the data were collected by, and based on, Poor Law Unions, so the reference to 'Bristol' meant the area covered by the Bristol Corporation of the Poor, and this was essentially the ancient urban core, within the boundaries established in 1373. By the 1840s the built up area had expanded significantly, and new neighbourhoods were included within either the Clifton Union or the Bedminster Union. All this posed a considerable problem for anyone wishing to construct reliable mortality figures for urban Bristol, because both the Clifton and Bedminster Unions embraced parishes well beyond the built up area. Figures limited to the old, overcrowded inner city of Bristol inevitably gave a distorted picture of the city as a whole. Clifton had the lowest rate of all the places in the Registrar General's table, and therefore a combined figure would not have looked so bad.

Substantial and sustainable improvement in mortality required two things: a reliable supply of clean water and effective means of removing domestic waste products. Neither of these was easy to achieve in the political context of the time. Among the many difficulties faced by public health reformers in Bristol in the 1840s was the fact that the town council was controlled by the Tories, who were disinclined to increase the rates burden on local property owners. They were, for example, unwilling to commit to a municipal water supply, relying instead on the privately owned Bristol Waterworks Company, which was established in 1846. The council was also unenthusiastic about adopting the Public Health Act, 1848, but the city's high mortality made it vulnerable to central imposition of a local board of health. The council therefore initiated the process itself, and this led to the third survey of conditions in the city, conducted by George Clark on behalf of the General Board of Health in February of 1850. His report of more than 200 pages went into great detail but essentially reiterated and confirmed the findings of William Kay and Henry De la Beche. The upshot was that in August 1851 Bristol town council was constituted as a local board of health (in practice the day to day work was carried out by a committee of the council). This set in train a twenty year programme of sewer construction that began in 1853, but even by the end of the century not everyone in Bristol had piped water or mains sewerage.

REFERENCES

1. Flinn, M, 'Introduction' in Chadwick, E, Report on the Sanitary Condition of the Labouring Population of Great Britain, (1842) Edinburgh: Edinburgh University Press, 1965, p16
2. Ibid, p4
3. Latimer, J, Annals of Bristol in the Nineteenth Century, Bristol, 1887, p312
4. Klein, R 'Edwin Chadwick 1800-1890' in Barker, P (ed) Founders of the Welfare State, London: Heinemann, 1984, p8
5. Ibid, p13
6. Finer, S E, The Life and Times of Sir Edwin Chadwick, London: Methuen, 1952, p234. and also in Lewis, RA, Edwin Chadwick and the Public health Movement 1832-1854, London: Longmans, Green and Co, 1952, p 887
7. Kay was also a Conservative member of the town council, 1842-44, and alderman 1844-50, Bush, G, Bristol and Its Municipal Government 1820-1851, Bristol: Bristol Record Society, 1976, p241. He was also secretary of the Bristol Association for Improving the Public Health. According to Lewis, op cit, p 86, Chadwick commissioned a series of reports from friends of public health reform in a number of towns, and it is probable that Kay's report arose in this way.
8. Kay, W, 'Report on the Sanatory [sic] Condition of Clifton', in Appendix - part I to the Second Report of the Commissioners for Inquiring into the State of Large Towns and Populous Districts, London; HMSO, 1845, accessed at: http://parlipapers.chadwyck.co.uk/marketing/index.jsp (October 2013)
9. De la Beche, Sir H, Report on the State of Bristol and Other Large Towns, London: HMSO, 1845. The commissioners each took responsibility for a series of local investigations. De la Beche also visited Bath, Frome, Swansea, Merthyr and Brecon. Playfair's towns were in Lancashire but for reasons unknown he also worked on the Bristol study. De la Beche was a noted geologist and palaeontologist, and first director of the geological survey of Great Britain. Playfair was a chemist who went on to have a political career as a Liberal and became baron Playfair in 1892.
10. Finer, op cit p234
11. Green, J Account of Recent Improvements in the Drainage and Sewerage of Bristol, Paper presented to the Institute of Civil Engineers, 8 February 1848, London: Clowes and Sons, p3-4
12. Eveleigh, op cit, pp12-15
13. Clark, G, Report to the General Board of Health, on a preliminary inquiry into the sewerage, drainage and supply of water, and of the sanitary condition of the inhabitants of the city and county of Bristol, 1850, BRO B1000, p85
14. De la Beche op cit p19
15. Frazer, op cit p69. See also Whitfield, M The Bristol Microscopists and the Cholera Epidemic of 1849, Bristol: ALHA, 2011
16. De la Beche, op cit, p49
17. Ibid, p16

THE BRISTOL MEDICO-HISTORICAL SOCIETY
Programme 2012-2016

Sept 2012
Mr Vincent Marmion : The medical aspects of the 1904 Mission to Tibet - the Younghusband expedition
Prof Gordon Stirrat: Medical Fraud – Causes and Consequences

Dec 2012
Mike Ruscoe: Syphilis and Shakespeare.
Charles Lewin: Edward Lear and his Health

March 2013
Ms Katie Hall (Med Student): Shell Shock, Septimus Smith and Mrs Dalloway.
John Harcup: Florence Nightingale and the Malvern Waters

June 2013
Dr Brandon Lush: The MRC - a cautionary tale
Prof Paul Goddard - the first Junior Doctor Strike.

Sept 2013
Dr Martin Crosfill: Francis Galton - a passion for measurement
Dr Peter Carpenter (in lieu of Ms Katherine Conlon): a history of ECT.

Dec 2013
Roger Rolls: Physic with a fizz - the medical history of soft drinks
Mike Whitfield: The first Baptist Missionary to India - Dr Thomas from Gloucestershire

March 2014
Tom Nutting: (Med Student): Fin-de-siècle male hysteria
Jonathan Bird: The kindest cut of all: A history of psycho-surgery at the Burden Institute

June 2014
Prof Dunn: Fetal Compression and the recognition of fetal deformation 1960 - 81
Prof Francis Duck - Edith and Florence Stoney: X-ray Pioneers.

Sept 2014
Dr Musgrave: a snapshot of skeletal and oral health in Minoan Crete.
Mr Gilison: The risks of operations on royalty and near-royalty

Dec 2014
Dr Burns Cox - Life of a colonial Medical Officer in North Borneo 1963-5.
Dr Stevens - Chlorosis - life and death of an illness

March 2015
Ellie Granger (Med Student): Schizophrenia and philosophy 35.
Greg Oxenham (Med Student):- Tuberculosis and the Operatic Heroine.

June 2015
- Conflict at the Children's hospital
Mike Whitfield - Dr Eubulus Williams
Judith Franklin - Eliza Dunbar Nil.

Sept 2015
Dr Bruno Bubna-Kasteliz: a Short history of Old Age Pensions
P Carpenter: Inebriacy in Bristol Typeset

Dec 2015
Prof Dunn: Childbed fever - its rise and fall.
Dr Y Wiley - stories from Broadmoor tribunals.

April 2016
Professor Tom Baskett... The Pill and the Pope

June 2016
Professor Peter Malpass: The Public Health of Victorian Bristol